ADVANCE PRAISE FOR *MOTIVATIONAL INTERVIEWING IN HIV CARE*

"A comprehensive, well-referenced handbook that is helpful for any practitioner interested in incorporating MI into their HIV practice. This book covers not only the basics of performing MI, but also provides specific examples illustrating methods to help patients with HIV infection engage in care, adhere to their antiretroviral regimen, and effectively deal with substance use. The experts who have authored each chapter provide an evidence-based approach with ample examples of demonstration projects which have successfully leveraged MI techniques to help patients with HIV infection succeed with their care."

—Jamie Riddell IV, MD,
Clinical Professor,
Division of Infectious Diseases,
Michigan Medicine,
University of Michigan

"The HIV epidemic is no longer front-page news with the transformation of the infection from an acute, lethal illness to a chronic disease. But with all of the successful pharmacological interventions, there continues to be over 40,000 new infections per year in the United States and millions throughout the world. Thus the need for prevention and treatment continues to require approaches that help identify those at risk, and those already infected. Barriers to identification of infection and engagement into treatment, and maintenance of adherence to lifesaving treatment require population focused clinical interventions. *Motivational Interviewing in HIV Care* provides an excellent source to help meet this clinical need. Using the structure of MI, each chapter addresses a specific aspect of the continuum of care. This book is accessible to readers new to MI as well as those with a strong background who can utilize MI to treat patients with HIV. Chapters provide evidence-based interventions for patients including adolescents and young adults. Strategies for increasing engagement in care and incorporation of the treatment of substance use disorders into the continuum of HIV care are especially important given the high risk for minority adolescents. Overall, every behavioral health and primary care provider would find this book clinically useful, especially with patients for whom treatment is problematic."

—Marshall Forstein, MD,
Associate Professor of Psychiatry Harvard Medical School,
Vice Chair for Education and Training,
Cambridge Health Alliance

"*Motivational Interviewing in HIV Care* nicely illustrates that engaging patients in meaningful conversations while examining personal health behavior adjustments can improve adherence to pre-exposure prophylaxis (PrEP) and antiretroviral therapy

(ART) while offering healthy lifestyle choices. The "Stages in Learning Motivational Interviewing" chapter assists practitioners in their assessment of the time, commitment and training needed to become proficient in this method of care. The reader gains a thorough understanding of the benefits, challenges, and ethical implications surrounding the MI counseling method. This book offers practical methods that can be used alone or in conjunction with other modalities to develop positive patient relationships and treatment outcomes."

—John W. Mellors, MD,
Chief, Division of Infectious Diseases,
Endowed Chair for Elimination of HIV and AIDS,
University of Pittsburgh School of Medicine

"The editors of this book, along with the expert authors, have brought together the broad literature on MI and skillfully applied it to the HIV continuum of care. Beginning with a thorough orientation, the text provides clinicians with an understanding of the key elements of MI, applies MI to a variety of clinical scenarios, and offers case examples to highlight interviewing techniques. The remaining chapters provide evidence and potential applications of MI to the entire HIV continuum, including linkage and engagement in care as well as medication adherence, and then expand to address special populations, HIV co-morbidities, and several ethical considerations. This book provides a valuable resource to any HIV practitioner wishing to learn about MI, or improve their existing skills with patients."

—Sybil Hosek, PhD,
Clinical Psychologist/Director of Research,
Department of Psychiatry,
Stroger Hospital of Cook County, Chicago, IL

MOTIVATIONAL INTERVIEWING IN HIV CARE

Edited by
Antoine Douaihy, MD

Professor of Psychiatry and Medicine

University of Pittsburgh School of Medicine

Senior Academic Director of Addiction Medicine Services

University of Pittsburgh Medical Center-Western Psychiatric Hospital

K. Rivet Amico, PhD

Associate Professor

Department of Health Behavior and Health Education

School of Public Health

University of Michigan

OXFORD
UNIVERSITY PRESS

OXFORD
UNIVERSITY PRESS

Oxford University Press is a department of the University of Oxford. It furthers
the University's objective of excellence in research, scholarship, and education
by publishing worldwide. Oxford is a registered trade mark of Oxford University
Press in the UK and certain other countries.

Published in the United States of America by Oxford University Press
198 Madison Avenue, New York, NY 10016, United States of America.

Library of Congress Cataloging-in-Publication Data
Names: Douaihy, Antoine, 1965– editor.
Title: Motivational interviewing in HIV care / [edited by] Antoine Douaihy, K. Rivet Amico.
Description: New York, NY : Oxford University Press, [2020] |
Includes bibliographical references and index. |
Identifiers: LCCN 2019039309 (print) | LCCN 2019039310 (ebook) |
ISBN 9780190619954 (paperback) | ISBN 9780190619961 (updf) |
ISBN 9780190619978 (epub) | ISBN 9780190619985 (online) |
ISBN 9780190619992 (Wrapper online)
Subjects: LCSH: HIV-positive persons—Counseling of. |
HIV-positive persons—Care. | Motivational interviewing.
Classification: LCC RC606.6 .M68 2020 (print) |
LCC RC606.6 (ebook) | DDC 616.97/92—dc23
LC record available at https://lccn.loc.gov/2019039309
LC ebook record available at https://lccn.loc.gov/2019039310

9 8 7 6 5 4 3 2 1

Printed by Marquis, Canada

Contents

Section I. Orientation to Motivational Interviewing and the Continuum of HIV Care in Practice

Section II. Applications of Motivational Interviewing: Intervening in the Continuum of HIV Care

Section III. Applications of Motivational Interviewing in Addressing
Comorbid Conditions

Section IV. Implementation of Motivational Interviewing

Section V. Ethics

Foreword

It is a genuine delight to introduce this volume. Our journeys since introducing motivational interviewing (MI) in the 1980s have included the HIV field. We have worked in African countries, trained many practitioners, observed the ravages of poverty and sickness, and met the most remarkable practitioners trying to use MI to engage people with HIV in urban and remote rural settings. Too little of this experience has been collected and shared. This volume closes the gap, with a thoroughness and clinical wisdom that we much admire. The authors know this field intimately.

This book provides an update on the state of play in the HIV field more broadly and then drills down on exactly how MI might help in various everyday scenarios, engagement being one of the most prominent. Examples of MI-consistent consultations reveal quite clearly how a simple conversation can impact outcome in powerful ways.

The challenges of engaging and helping hard-to-reach people are widespread. Clearly, MI is not a miracle method, and there are challenges in helping practitioners to adjust their practice to a more collaborative approach. Yet the evidence for using MI in this field is persuasive. If you are new to the HIV field or already a busy clinician wanting to make a difference, this volume is a welcome resource. We thank the authors for a wise and wonderful contribution to the field.

Stephen Rollnick, PhD
Honorary Distinguished Professor
School of Medicine, Cardiff University
Wales, United Kingdom
William R. Miller, PhD
Emeritus Distinguished Professor of Psychology and Psychiatry
University of New Mexico

Preface

Motivational interviewing (MI), an empirically based approach originally developed by William R. Miller and Stephen Rollnick, represents both a clinical presence ("spirit") and a set of pragmatic skills and strategies designed to help people change and sustain health promoting behaviors. MI, rooted in the Rogerian person-centered therapy and humanistic psychology, is goal-oriented and focuses fundamentally on understanding the person's perspectives rather than framing problems from a practitioner's mindset. MI fosters a constructive practitioner–patient relationship and leads to better outcomes for patients. MI respects patients' ambivalence about making changes and strategically strengthens motivation for change. There has been an explosion of research evidence supporting the efficacy and effectiveness of MI-based approaches across health-related conditions, including HIV. For service and care providers of HIV-related services, engaging and supporting individuals living with HIV are critically important in closing the gaps in the HIV care continuum. People living with HIV manage daily medication, quarterly or bi-annual care visits, and, in many cases, high levels of HIV stigma with new diagnoses in the United States and worldwide disproportionately impacting marginalized communities. Medical, social, and community-based practitioners engage with patients often and risk promoting disengagement when services are not grounded in a spirit of humility and person-centeredness. MI has increasingly been used to facilitate supportive, candid discussions between patients and HIV service practitioners. The individually tailored nature of MI empowers patients to learn to identify and prioritize their own problems, take appropriate action on their terms, and enlist the support needed to solve these problems in collaboration with healthcare practitioners and concerned significant others. This book, inspired by the spirit of MI, reflects the significant advances in research and clinical practice of MI in HIV care. It integrates our understanding and experiences of MI with the evidence-based recommendations of other clinicians and scientists in HIV care. MI is clearly gaining a momentum in the field of HIV, and we are fortunate enough to share a collaborative project that brought together researchers and practitioners who have made significant contributions to the growth and development of MI in HIV care.

We hope this book will propel practitioners to learn and train in MI and eventually integrate it as a tool in their therapeutic toolbox. Practitioners working with people living with HIV will appreciate the tremendous amount of therapeutic experiences, clinical illustrations, research applications, and invaluable insights shared in this book and will empower them to find ways of integrating MI into their clinical practice. Additionally, we hope this volume will inspire researchers to develop innovative approaches to understanding MI change processes and implementation strategies for MI interventions in HIV care.

This book is arranged into five parts. Part I is intended to lay the foundation for the application of MI in HIV care, provide an overview of MI, and discuss the spirit of the MI approach and its therapeutic processes, skills, and strategies. The second part contains four chapters devoted to the applications of MI along the HIV continuum of care. Part III reviews the applications of MI in addressing social determinants of HIV outcomes. Part IV addresses the processes of learning and training in MI, implementing it, incorporating it into technology, and integrating it with other treatment modalities. Part V focuses on ethical challenges in applying MI in HIV care.

Acknowledgments

I want to express my regard and deep appreciation to the outstanding community of colleagues of the Motivational Interviewing Network of Trainers, known as MINT, and the HIV field in the United States and internationally. You inspire me. This book was made possible because of the work and influence of pioneers in the field of motivational interviewing, Bill Miller and Steve Rollnick. I also wish to express my heartfelt appreciation to all the contributors who have shared their work and invaluable insights. Finally, this manuscript could not have been completed without the help and wonderful support of Andrea Knobloch from Oxford University Press.

Specific thanks to all the research teams, participants, advocates, and communities who have contributed so much to leading the charge in making HIV care humble, responsive, and person-facing K. Rivet Amico.

Antoine Douaihy

About the Editors

Antoine Douaihy, MD, is Professor of Psychiatry and Medicine at the University of Pittsburgh School of Medicine, Senior Academic Director of Addiction Medicine Services, Director of the Addiction Psychiatry Fellowship at Western Psychiatric Hospital of the University of Pittsburgh Medical Center (UPMC), and Co-Director of Tobacco Treatment Service at UPMC. He has a well-established record of clinical, leadership, and research expertise in substance use disorders (SUDs) and SUDs co-occurring with psychiatric disorders, psychology of behavior change, motivational interviewing, and HIV. He is a member of the Motivational Interviewing Network of Trainers (MINT) and has a substantial experience in training and disseminating motivational interviewing and brief interventions in HIV care and other medical and psychiatric settings. Dr. Douaihy has a well-established record of leadership and expertise in conducting clinical trials having served and serves as a PI, Co-PI and Co-I on NIAAA, NIMH, NIDA, HRSA, SAMHSA, and industry sponsored grants.

K. Rivet Amico, PhD, is Associate Professor in the Department of Health Behavior and Health Education, School of Public Health, University of Michigan. Dr. Amico is an active contributor in the areas of HIV-prevention and treatment, social-behavioral theory development, intervention implementation, evaluation, and measurement. Her research includes work with engagement in HIV care, TB, and drug-resistant TB prevention and treatment, Pre-Exposure Prophylaxis (PrEP), social and behavioral factors influencing participants in clinical trials, and measures development. Dr. Amico's investment is largely in applied, practical work, that can effectively advance the reach and quality of care and prevention services available domestically and internationally. Dr. Amico has strong interests in research design, implementation science, program evaluation, and community capacity building.

Contributors

K. Rivet Amico, PhD
Department of Health Behavior and
Health Education, School of Public
Health, University of Michigan
Ann Arbor, MI, USA

Priyanka Amin, MD
Western Psychiatric Hospital
Pittsburgh, PA, USA

Pierre N. Azzam, MD
University of Pittsburgh School of
Medicine
Pittsburgh, PA, USA

Claire Becker
University of Pittsburgh School of
Medicine
Pittsburgh, PA, USA

Isra Black, PhD
York Law School, The University of York
York, England

Robert Bolan, MD
Los Angeles Gay and Lesbian
Community Service Center
Los Angeles, CA, USA

Steve Bradley-Bull
UNC Center for AIDS Research (CFAR)
Chapel Hill, NC, USA

Maurice Bulls, MEd
Behavior Change Consulting
Royal Oak, Michigan, USA

Breana Uhrig Castonguay, MPH
UNC Center for AIDS Research (CFAR)
Chapel Hill, NC, USA

Sofie L. Champassak, PhD
Center for Stress and Healthy Aging
San Diego, CA, USA

Larry Chang, MD
Johns Hopkins Medicine
Baltimore, MD, USA

Jin Cheng, MD
University of Pittsburgh Medical Center
Pittsburg, PA, USA

Sharon Connor, PharmD
University of Pittsburgh
Pittsburgh, PA, USA

Sarah Dewing, PhD
South African Medical Research
Council
Cape Town, South Africa

Antoine Douaihy, MD
University of Pittsburgh School of
Medicine
Pittsburgh, PA, USA

Risa Flynn
LGBT Center
Los Angeles, CA, USA

Lisa Forsberg, PhD
Oxford Uehiro Centre for Practical Ethics
Oxford, England

Linda R. Frank, PhD
Graduate School of Public Health
University of Pittsburgh
Pittsburgh, PA, USA

Carol Golin, MD
University of North Carolina–Chapel
Hill School of Medicine
UNC Center of AIDS Research
Chapel Hill, NC, USA

Catherine Grodensky, MPH
Duke University Sanford School of
Public Policy
Chapel Hill, NC, USA

Lisa Hightow-Weidman, MD
University of North Carolina School of
Medicine
Chapel Hill, NC, USA

**Marcia M. Holstad, PhD, FNP-BC,
FAANP, FAAN**
Nell Hodgson Woodruff School of
Nursing
Emory Center for AIDS
Atlanta, GA, USA

Heidi Hutton, PhD
Associate Professor of Psychiatry &
Behavioral Sciences
Johns Hopkins Medicine
Baltimore, MD, USA

Megan Mueller Johnson, MA
University of Michigan School of
Public Health
Ann Arbor, MI, USA

Shriya Kaneriya, MD
Western Psychiatric Hospital
Pittsburgh, PA, USA

Kelly Amy Knudtson, MPH
Program Manager, Infectious Diseases,
UNC-Chapel Hill
Chapel Hill, NC, USA

Liu yi Lin, MD
Western Psychiatric Hospital
Pittsburgh, PA, USA

Gordon Liu, MD
University of Pittsburgh School of
Medicine
Pittsburgh, PA, USA

David A. Martinez, PhD
University of San Francisco, School of
Nursing and Health Professions
San Francisco, CA, USA

Cathy Mathews, PhD
South African Medical Research
Council
Cape Town, South Africa

Riddhi Modi, MBBS, MPH
University of Alabama at Birmingham
Birmingham, AL, USA

Sylvie Naar, PhD
Center for Translational Behavioral
Science
Florida State University
Tallahassee, FL, USA

Ramakrishna Prasad, MD, MPH
Founder & Director, PCMH Restore
Health; Vice President, AFPI Karnataka
Bangalore, Karnataka, India

Laramie Smith, PhD
University of California, San Diego
San Diego, CA, USA

Peter Veldkamp, MD
University of Pittsburgh School of
Medicine
Pittsburgh, PA, USA

Hanna K. Welch, PharmD
University of Louisiana Monroe College
of Pharmacy
Monroe, LA, USA

Motivational Interviewing in HIV Care

SECTION I
ORIENTATION TO MOTIVATIONAL INTERVIEWING AND THE CONTINUUM OF HIV CARE IN PRACTICE

1 Overview of Motivational Interviewing

Shriya Kaneriya, Antoine Douaihy, and Peter Veldkamp

Conversations about change are embedded in every day interactions between people. The various shades of language used in these exchanges, both consciously and subconsciously, influence behaviors, particularly an individual's motivation to change them. Behavior and lifestyle choices have meaningful implications for a person's health and are integral to managing chronic conditions like HIV illness. Thus, healthcare practitioners across all disciplines regularly find themselves engaging in change conversations, hoping to encourage patients to reduce harmful behaviors and inspire engagement with positive ones. However, anyone who has ever considered making a behavioral change or tried to convince another to do so would likely acknowledge that changing behaviors is not an easy task. Despite the best of intentions, it can often feel instinctual to lecture or plead, leading to ineffective conversations that can often become detrimental to the therapeutic relationship. Motivational interviewing (MI) offers a more constructive, egalitarian way to navigate such challenges and help patients find motivation within themselves to make health behavior changes.

WHAT IS MOTIVATIONAL INTERVIEWING?

In the third edition of *Motivational Interviewing: Helping People Change*, Miller and Rollick[1] offer the following definitions of MI, each with evolving technical complexity to allow accessibility for both laypersons and healthcare practitioners:

1. "A collaborative conversation style for strengthening a person's own motivation and commitment to change."[1p12]
2. "A person-centered counseling style for addressing the common problems of ambivalence about change."[1p24]
3. "A collaborative, goal-directed style of communication with particular attention to the language of change. It is designed to strengthen personal motivation for, and

commitment to, a specific goal by eliciting and exploring the person's own reasons for change within an atmosphere of acceptance and compassion."[1p29]

MI is a practical, brief, and evidence-based approach that takes into consideration how difficult it is to make behavioral changes. Ambivalence represents a patient's experience of simultaneously feeling conflicted (two ways) about changing one's behavior, for example, concurrently wanting to make a change while also feeling reluctant to do so. Within clinical encounters and MI approach, ambivalence is conceptualized as patient expressions in favor of change ("change talk"), which often co-exist with patient expressions in favor of wanting to keep the status quo ("sustain talk"; e.g., "I know I need to take my HIV medications, but they remind me of being positive!"). Ambivalence is defined as a "normal step on the road to change."[1p157] In essence, MI is about "arranging conversations so people talk themselves into change based on their own values and interests."[1p] Inherent in this method is an attention and appreciation for the language of change and the way attitudes are not only reflected, but also actively shaped by speech.

Core Communication Skills

There are three core communication skills that are part of MI: informing, asking, and listening.[2] These are widely applicable skills that can be modulated to match the style of communication being used at a particular time with a patient. *Informing* entails providing factual knowledge about a medical diagnosis, treatment, testing result, prognosis, or management recommendation. *Asking* entails developing an understanding of a patient's problems and perspectives through open-ended questions. This type of inquiry is in contrast to close-ended questions that elicit "yes/no" answers and are often used to determine a medical course of action later objectively relayed to the patient. *Listening* entails an active effort to understand the experiences, feelings, and meanings that can be drawn from what the patient is saying. Instead of a simple head nod or a verbalized "Uh huh" or "I see," active listening can be demonstrated through the use of reflective statements, a skill that will be discussed in more detail in Chapter 3.

Core Communication Styles

There are three core communications styles: directing, following, and guiding. It can be useful to think about helping conversations as lying on a spectrum. At one end is the *directing* style, where the practitioner is the expert who provides information and instruction, such as how to take a medication properly. The communication implied in this style is "I know what you should do, and here is how to do it." At the opposite end of the spectrum is the *following* style, where the practitioner is a good listener trying to understand the patient's perspective without interjecting his or her own agenda. The communication implied in this style is "I trust your own wisdom, I will stay with you, and I will let you work this out in your own way." In the middle of the spectrum is the *guiding* style, where the practitioner seeks to skillfully be both a good listener and offer expertise when needed. MI is an example of a guiding communication style. Different patient encounters lend themselves to different communication styles, with no single one better than the others. All three styles are important, and the art of clinical practice exists in being able to identify which style is appropriate to a situation and how to flexibly shift between them.

THE SPIRIT OF MOTIVATIONAL INTERVIEWING

To be effective, MI goes beyond simply using the technical component of skills and processes (discussed in Chapter 2). There is a fundamental relational aspect. In MI practice, therapists' must negotiate this delicate balance of relational and technical skills to navigate the MI session focusing on helping the patient explore and resolve ambivalence in the direction of behavior change.[3] MI is a clinical way of being with another person who is nonjudgmental and based on compassion, respect, and empathy. It is this humanistic quality that highlights the "spirit" of MI[4] without which the technical intervention could not be effective. MI is not a trick to manipulate individuals into doing what they do not want to do.[5] It is rather a meeting of minds and hearts, focused together toward a common goal for positive change. The essential spirit of MI is grounded in a sense of genuine curiosity about the patient's world and the prioritization of the value and agency of individual persons over the solely rational and empirical. The spirit of MI is at the foundation of every MI conversation and comprises of four key elements in the acronym PACE (Table 1.1): partnership, acceptance, compassion, and evocation. One need not be fully proficient in these elements to begin practicing MI. Engaging in the practice itself can teach the spirit of an open mind and heart.[2]

Partnership (vs. Authority/Confrontation)

In MI, the relationship between the practitioner and patient is that of an equal partnership. MI is done "for" and "with" someone, not "to" or "on" them. Goals are focused on whatever specific behavior change the patient wishes to make. The role of the practitioner is to explore the patients' perspective and experience to understand the circumstances that motivated them to seek care and to evoke their underlying reasons to change. This type of relationship contrasts with more traditional approaches, which are based on the practitioner assuming the role of expert and the patient becoming a passive recipient of information. In this model, the expert is at times confronting the patient and imposing his or her opinions on an unhealthy behavior and how it should be changed. Such an approach undermines patients' undisputed expertise on themselves.

Table 1.1. The Spirit of MI: Four Key Elements

	Basic Language Primer Associations
Partnership	"We are going to work together."
Acceptance	"I value who you are and respect your decision."
Compassion	"I care about you and want to understand your experience."
Evocation	"With all the things that get in your way, what makes you determined to change?"

Alternatively, the collaborative spirit of MI helps facilitate rapport and trust in the helping relationship, a crucial element that is challenging to achieve in a more hierarchical approach. Establishing partnership involves learning to be attuned to the subtleties of verbal and nonverbal dialogue and recognizing their significance in setting the tone for the therapeutic relationship. Partnership does not mean that the practitioners must automatically agree with the patient's opinions and choices. It does, however, require them to develop awareness of their own perspective and how it relates with that of the patient. Although two individuals may see things differently, the therapeutic process is focused on a mutual understanding and not the practitioner always being right.

Here's how the collaborative style can be reinforced:

- "May I discuss with you my perspective on the importance of taking antiretroviral therapy for your HIV illness? We could review different treatment regimen options, and you can decide what you feel most comfortable taking."
- "You raise important concerns about your drinking and its impact on your taking medications. You expressed desire to reduce your drinking. We can review some options to help you do it."

Acceptance

Accepting the patient means that the practitioner recognizes and respects all that a person brings to a partnership. Acceptance does not require that the practitioner personally approve of a person's behaviors or choices. However, the practitioner must accept them. Acceptance consists of four elements: (i) absolute worth, (ii) accurate empathy, (iii) autonomy support, and (iv) affirmation.

Accurate empathy is an active, genuine interest in understanding how every person sees the world. Empathy is not the same as sympathy. It is rather the ability to appreciate patients frame of reference and validate that their perspective is worthwhile. Empathy can be communicated to patients with the use of thoughtful reflections. The opposite of this concept is the imposition of one's own values and perception at the price of dismissing the patient's perception as misguided or insignificant.

Absolute worth is acknowledging and respecting the inherent value and potential of every individual human being. Ultimately, everyone is on a journey trying to figure out who they are, where they are going, and how they are going to get there. This aspect of acceptance assumes that no person is entirely devoid of goodness or trustworthiness. Discovering these inner qualities is a critical part of behavior change. An attitude of unconditional acceptance toward others not only allows practitioners to stay open to a person's intrinsic goodness, but also helps patients who feel they are lacking in some way believe that they too possess this quality. The opposite of this attitude is judgment. People can become immobilized when they experience themselves as unacceptable. In contrast, when people feel accepted and learn to accept themselves, they are far more likely to become free to implement and sustain the change they seek.

A patient who was recently diagnosed with HIV has difficulty opening up about his feelings of shame. Some ways demonstrating acceptance of the patient's struggle include:

- "You are in a lot of pain and feel so embarrassed about sharing your struggle coping with being HIV positive."
- "What's like for you to go through the pain of coping with being HIV positive?"

Autonomy support is honoring each person's irrevocable right and capacity for self-determination and the freedom to be who they are and choose what they will become. MI fosters self-efficacy and builds on the principle that patients themselves are the agents of change.[6] This is not only empowering to the individuals, but also gives them responsibility for their actions. The opposite of autonomy support is authoritative control and coercion, such as telling a patient "you can" do something. Such statements of curbing choice generally backfire. They incite resistance and a desire to assert one's freedom. To shift toward autonomy support, practitioners must let go of the burdensome idea that they should, or can, make people change. This concept recognizes that there is no single "right way" to change.

Some reflective statements illustrating autonomy support:

- "It is up to you to decide whether you want to stop or reduce your drinking."
- "Since you are conflicted about staying on antiretroviral therapy (ART), we can review the pros and cons of taking ART and you can decide whether you want to pursue treatment or not."

Affirmation is seeking to acknowledge a person's strengths and efforts to maintain behavior change. The opposite of affirmation is concentrating efforts on identifying what is wrong with people and telling them how to fix it. Statements of affirmation remind patients that their experiences are being heard and that they already possess the resilience needed to face their challenges. In the midst of present hardship, it can sometimes be difficult to remember one's past successes.

- "You have dealt with so many challenges getting in the way of your adhering to ART and HIV treatment and you managed to follow through with treatment and achieve an undetectable viral load and better quality of life living with HIV illness."
- "You have demonstrated a considerable resilience that helped you manage your HIV illness very well."

Compassion

Compassion is a deliberate commitment to actively promote another's welfare and prioritize his or her needs over one's own. This perspective extends the meaning of compassion beyond the emotional response of being moved by another's suffering and feeling the desire to relieve it. While partnership, acceptance, and evocation can be used in other professional settings to pursue self-interest, the spirit of compassion distinguishes the therapeutic relationship and ensures that one's intentions come from a pure place.

Evocation (Drawing Out)

Evocation is characterized by the way the practitioner draws out a person's own thoughts and ideas. This method diverges from traditional approaches of collecting patient information, relying on close-ended questions, and imposing opinions. In MI, the process of evocation is rooted in the belief that lasting motivation and commitment to change is most powerful and durable when the patients discover their own reasons and determination to change. Intrinsic motivation can be cultivated through collaborative engagement with a person's experiences and perspective.

The practitioner's role is to elicit the patients' motivation and capacity for change, not to tell them what to do or why they should do it. However, this can be a rather difficult role to practice for even most well-intentioned people in the healthcare field. It is both a natural and common feeling to want desperately to help someone by stepping in and "fixing" a patient's problem. This gut reaction is what is referred to as the "the righting reflex." Learning how to curb one's righting reflex is a fundamental aspect of learning and practicing MI. Telling patients why and how to make behavior changes has been shown to be ineffective in both helping them feel better and making health-related behavior change. It can also be damaging to the therapeutic relationship and push patients to engage in even more unhealthy behavior due to the pressure placed on them to make changes they weren't quite ready to make.

Some ways to illustrate the evocation component of the MI spirit include:

- "In what ways do you believe your HIV illness has affected your life and physical health?"
- "You have been so disciplined in managing your HIV illness and taking ART consistently, what are the driving forces that made you decide to take charge of your health?"
- "What sort of strategies do you believe would be helpful for you to use so you prevent missing any doses of your medication?"

MI is a collaborative conversation about change that rests not on the flaws of an individual, but in the power of harnessing his or her strengths. The approach understands that readiness to change exists on a continuum and that ambivalence is a normal part of the change process. Practitioners should learn to guard against their righting reflex and desire to "fix" patients by telling them what to do. Individuals are more likely to be persuaded into behavior change by what they hear themselves articulate rather than by what they are told. The primary purpose of MI is to strengthen motivation for change from within through a spirit of partnership, acceptance, compassion, and evocation (Figure 1.1). This spirit of MI is carried by a guiding style of communication where practitioners are able to adjust between core communication skills to meet patients at their unique level of motivation. Integrating the practice of MI into clinical settings can more effectively help motivate patients to choose healthy lifestyle behaviors. The next chapters will describe in more detail the method of MI, including four critical skills and how they can be used to navigate between the four processes of MI.

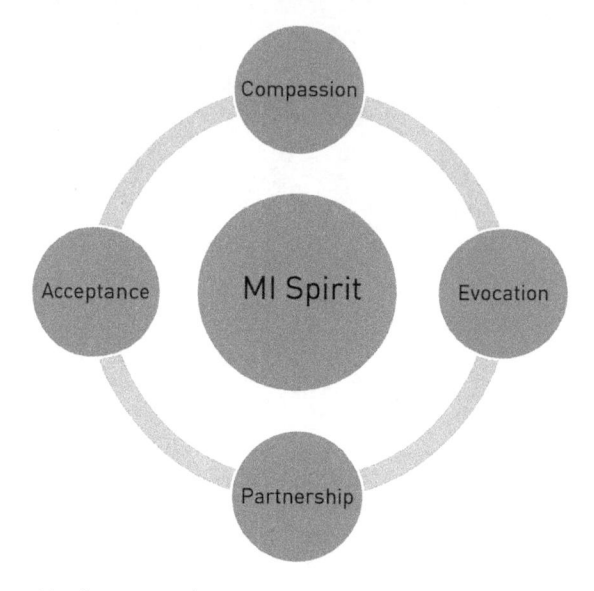

FIGURE 1.1. The spirit of motivational interviewing.

REFERENCES

1. Miller WR, Rollnick S. *Motivational Interviewing: Helping People Change.* 3rd ed. New York, NY: Guilford Press; 2013.
2. Douaihy A, Kelly TM, Gold MA, eds. *Motivational Interviewing: A Guide for Medical Trainees.* New York, NY: Oxford University Press; 2014.
3. Miller WR, Rose GS. Toward a theory of motivational interviewing. *Am Psychol.* 2009;64(6):527–537.
4. Miller WR, Rollnick S. *Motivational Interviewing: Preparing People for Change.* 2nd ed. New York, NY: Guildford Press; 2002.
5. Miller WR, Rollnick S. Ten things that motivational interviewing is not. *Behav Cogn Psychother.* 2009;37(2):129–140.
6. Resnicow K, McMaster F. Motivational Interviewing: moving from why to how with autonomy support. *Int J Behav Nutr Phys Act.* 2012;9:19. doi:10.1186/1479-5868-9-19

2 Motivational Interviewing Processes and Skills

Priyanka Amin, Antoine Douaihy, and Ramakrishna Prasad

Motivational interviewing (MI) is a person-centered approach with the primary goal of eliciting change talk. There are four key processes in MI: engaging, focusing, evoking, and planning.[1,2]

ENGAGING (RELATIONAL FOUNDATION)

Establishing and cultivating an engaging partnership with patients begins the moment the interaction starts. Engagement is conveyed by both nonverbal and verbal features of an interaction. Initial body language and nonverbal cues start this process. For example, making sure that you are seated at or below the patient with an open body posture, facing the patient, and making eye contact at the beginning of the encounter can help a patient feel more comfortable and at ease. The alternative, where the patient is placed in a physical position of less power, conveys a noncollaborative relationship. Similarly, meeting in a private space where patients feel safe opening up, without fear of others hearing what they are saying or passing judgment on them, conveys respect and placing a premium on the patient's comfort. Verbally, many of the core features of MI are intended to convey genuine engagement through reflection, probes, and an overall spirit that centers on the patient's own concerns and experiences. Monitoring verbal and nonverbal reactions to ensure a compassionate and respectful stance is fundamental to MI-based communication.

FOCUSING (COLLABORATIVELY DEVELOPING DIRECTION/STRATEGY)

After building rapport and engaging a patient, the next task is to set an agenda to help focus the clinical encounter ("strategic centering"). It is crucial that the patient be included in determining the agenda. If there are topics that you perceive to be of importance to discuss but the patient does not bring up for the agenda, an MI-adherent approach to addressing these topics would be to ask permission, such as "I wonder whether you would be willing to discuss condom use today. Would that be okay with you?" In MI, the goal is to help guide patients in the process of moving toward behavior change, while not taking too passive or too active of a role. As such, it is important to meet the patients where they are at in their behavior change and priorities when setting a direction for the encounter. It would not be reasonable to focus the conversation on strategies to be adherent to antiretroviral therapy if the patient is still ambivalent about the need to talk about them. Rather, it would be more productive to focus on exploring the ambivalence. At all times, patient autonomy should be respected.

EVOKING (DRAWING OUT INTRINSIC MOTIVATION)

A fundamental task of MI is to evoke from the patient his or her ambivalence about changing, reasons for change, and strategies for change. In this stage, the skills of MI such as reflective listening (discussed later in the chapter) become strategic in guiding the person in the direction of change by focusing on evoking "change talk." MI selectively elicits and reinforces change talk defined as expressing preparatory statements of desire, ability, reasons, and need for change (DARN) and mobilizing statements of commitment, activation, and taking steps (CAT). Preparatory talk means that the person is thinking about change and ready to consider it. Mobilizing talk indicates a movement toward change. "Sustain talk" is the opposite of change talk expressed by reasons and statements related to not wanting to change. The ratio of change talk to sustain talk that the person expresses is directly related to the probability of behavior change.[3] Here's an example of "change talk" in bold font and "sustain talk" in italic font:

I know I must take my antiretroviral regimen since I can live longer and have a better quality of life. *But taking the medication every day is such an inconvenience and I most of the time forget to take it and sometimes I have diarrhea from it and it interferes with my ability to stay focused at work and I don't want to talk it for the rest of my life.* **I realize that I need to stay healthy, so I can spend more quality time with my grandchildren and after all I don't want to die soon, I still have a lot to live for and enjoy in my life.**

Figure 2.1 provides an example of change talk (DARN-CAT) you may hear from patients who smoke cigarettes and who want to cut down or stop smoking.

Focusing on eliciting and strengthening change talk and not arguing against sustain talk can facilitate the process of change. This example demonstrates the process of evoking and inviting change talk, guiding the patient through expressing her own arguments and motivations for change, and avoiding the activation of the righting reflex. In standard medical practice, practitioners often provide information about the risks of continuing a behavior or emphasizing the benefits and importance of change with the intent of persuading the patient to move in the direction that the practitioners chose. Such statements like "It is very important that you take your medication" and "Changing your diet should be your top priority" elicit reactance and push back from the patient.[4,5] In contrast, MI uses an *elicit–provide–elicit* (E-P-E) framework in exchanging information. The practitioner first *elicits* the person's understanding and need for information about a specific topic (E) and then builds on the information and *provides* new

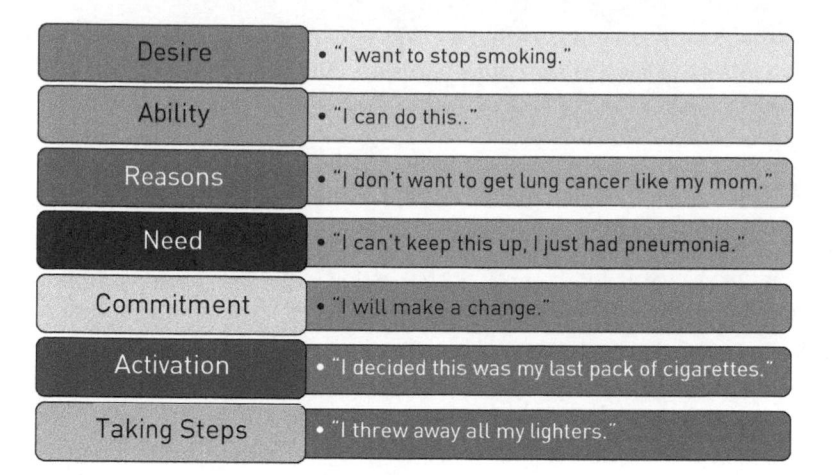

Desire	• "I want to stop smoking."
Ability	• "I can do this.."
Reasons	• "I don't want to get lung cancer like my mom."
Need	• "I can't keep this up, I just had pneumonia."
Commitment	• "I will make a change."
Activation	• "I decided this was my last pack of cigarettes."
Taking Steps	• "I threw away all my lighters."

FIGURE 2.1. Change talk statements: DARN-CAT.

information in a neutral manner (P), followed by *eliciting* what this information might mean for the patient and reflecting on the patient's view of what is offered (E).

This clinical encounter describes a patient-centered exchange maintaining collaboration, evocation, and respecting patient's autonomy while using a specific MI strategy of "rating ruler":

Patient: I'm really scared about my viral load going up. I am depressed.

Practitioner: You are terrified about your HIV illness not being well controlled and concerned about the consequences.

Patient: I don't want to suffer and die. I need to do something about it.

Practitioner: What do you believe is contributing to the increase in your viral load?

Patient: I have been cheating in the past few months and not taking my antiretroviral medication every day, and I'm concerned this is causing the increase.

Practitioner: You have been struggling with taking your medication every day.

Patient: Yes, and I know it is important to do it consistently; otherwise, it won't work.

Practitioner: You are making a valid point. How much is it important to you that you regain control over your HIV illness? Let's say on a scale of 0 to 10, 0 not important at all and 10 extremely important, top priority for you?

Patient: I think around 8.

Practitioner: It is highly important to you. How come it is an 8 not a 4?

Patient: You have discussed with me how much it is crucial to keep the viral load undetectable, so I would not suffer bad consequences from HIV.

Practitioner: What are you mostly concerned about?

Patient: Infections and other serious stuff that could compromise my functioning, my quality of life, and being able to take care of my children.

Practitioner: You want to prevent the impact of having your HIV illness uncontrolled, and you see the importance of taking your medication consistently. How do you feel about discussing the obstacles that get in the way of your taking your medication daily and review strategies to deal with them?

In this encounter, the patient is making the arguments for change and the practitioner is evoking them. We can help elicit change talk by understanding the reasons patients currently engage in certain behaviors and how they feel about their actions. Understanding a patient's motivations and values can also help evoke change talk. We will review the skills that foster evoking change talk later in this chapter.

PLANNING (BRIDGING TO CHANGE)

The final core process of MI is planning. This process involves refining a patient's commitment to change and discussing concrete action steps. It is important to consider what a reasonable action item is. For example, if a patient is planning to start a new exercise regimen, setting a goal of working out daily for an hour every day may be unrealistic if the patient is currently not exercising at all. Rather, discussing what the patient feels are reasonable goals that they can meet for their next clinical encounter may help them build confidence in the progress that they make. This also points to the importance of ongoing re-evaluation of action steps as well as of the direction of treatment.

Theoretically, the MI processes are somewhat linear and at the same time they are recursive and interwoven. *Engaging* continues throughout the whole encounter, *focusing* may change, and *evoking* can be initiated early in the encounter. MI is not considered MI without these 3 processes: engaging, focusing, and evoking. MI is considered MI when the style and "spirit" involve a person-centered empathic approach, when there is a specific target behavior for change that is the focus of the encounter, and when the practitioner is evoking the person's own motivations and ideas for change.

Fundamental to MI are the person-centered counseling skills that situate the communication strategies. These skills are used in a strategic manner to move the encounter in the direction of change throughout the MI processes. The skills are summarized in the mnemonic acronym OARS: open-ended questions, affirmation, reflection, and summaries.[1,2]

OPEN-ENDED QUESTIONS

We often fall into the trap of thinking that asking closed-ended questions will allow us to more rapidly obtain information. Asking open-ended questions allows our patients to describe their experience rather than us arriving to premature conclusions about how they are doing and what their concerns are. For example, asking a question such as "You take your medications daily, right?" is a leading question to which the patient may answer "yes" even if this is not the case.

In MI, starting with open-ended questions helps to engage patients and to evoke their intrinsic motivations and elicit change talk.

Examples of open-ended questions include

"Help me understand how you decided to seek treatment."
"What have you noticed after taking this HIV medication regimen?"
"How do you cope with your HIV illness?"

Examples of closed-ended question stems include

"Can you tell me why you came to treatment here?"
"Do you like taking your HIV medication regimen?"

In asking open-ended questions, using "why" in the question stem, such as "Why you are not taking your medication daily?" places patients on the defensive and decreases engagement, making it harder to work on behavioral change.

AFFIRMATIONS

We use affirmations in MI to acknowledge patients' prior successes and to recognize their strengths and skills. Affirmations are different from cheerleading or saying, "Great job!" or "I'm so proud of you!" as affirmations are specific and pertain directly to the patient. Specifics can include their efforts or their qualities. It is best to avoid using "I" in providing affirmations, as this shifts the focus of the affirmation away from the patient. Affirmations strengthen the therapeutic relationship. Using scare tactics and making people feel bad about their behaviors keep them more stuck and unable to change.

Examples of affirmations include

"You were resourceful in reaching out when you needed assistance."
"You have been very forthcoming and open about what you are going through."
"You have been able to stick to treatment and you are proud of your actions."

REFLECTIONS

Reflecting shows you are "actively listening" and engaged. Reflection is a crucial skill in MI. It appears easy, but it takes hard work to build. Learning to *think* reflectively takes hard work and time to build. It accompanies strong reflective listening. Reflective listening is meant to minimize any breakdowns in communication during the clinical encounter. Reflection is conceptualized as a form of hypothesis testing. As Miller and Rollnick[2] said, "good reflective listening tends to keep the person talking, exploring, and considering."

Reflections, particularly by practitioners who are just started learning and practicing MI, often begin with what we call "window dressing," such as "It sounds like . . . ," "It seems like . . . ," and "It looks like . . . ." Skilled practitioners often reframe their reflections in a more truncated form starting with a "you," such as "You are struggling with . . . ," leaving off the assumed "It sounds like . . ." or It seems like . . . ." There are two types of reflections: simple and complex. Simple reflections are a rewording of the emotion or content presented by a patient. While simple reflections may be helpful for initial engagement and rapport-building, they, by their nature, do little to advance the MI processes. In contrast, complex reflections can help facilitate conversation and increase the likelihood of change talk. Complex reflections add to the content or emotions that the patient presents. They infer meaning. They involve different levels of complexity and depth. Reflection of emotion is one of the deepest forms of empathic reflection. Double-sided reflections can be helpful for patients who are feeling ambivalent about changes. They can help guide the patient from a place of ambivalence to one where they are seeing discrepancies in their values versus current behaviors. Some examples of simple and complex reflections are as follows.

Patient: I am nervous that my CD4 count has gone down even though I've been taking my HIV medicine. I'm not sure if it is worth staying on medications, since it does not seem to be helping.

Simple reflection: You aren't sure if the medications are still helpful.

Complex reflection: You're scared that your health is worsening, and you are frustrated that you don't have control over it.

Complex reflection: You care so much about controlling your HIV illness, and you want to figure out the reasons for the changes in your blood work and whether the medications are working. You are also wondering what you could do to get a better control of your illness and live a healthier life.

In the previous complex reflection, there is amplification of expressed emotions as well as a reflection of underlying meaning. Patients may disagree with the underlying meaning in complex reflection: this is okay, as even when our reflections are not an accurate guess, if they come from a place of empathic listening, they allow patients to help clarify their experiences. A follow-up with a patient disagreeing with the reflective statement could be "Help me understand this from your viewpoint." As such, reflections can be evoking more from the patients. Varying the levels of reflection mobilizes the change process. At times, there are benefits to overstating or understating a reflection. An overstated reflection may cause a person to back away from their position or belief. An understated reflection may help a person to explore a deeper commitment to the position or belief. A deflection in the tone of the reflection keeps it as a reflection instead of turning into a question.

SUMMARIES

Summaries are helpful to consolidate information, to ensure that the practitioner has accurately heard the patient, which improves the therapeutic alliance; to highlight key points and organize information for the patient; to deepen the current conversation; and to transition topics.

There are three types of summaries: collecting, linking, and transitional.[1,2] Collecting summaries generally include a list of what information has been shared thus far. For example, if a patient is discussing their strengths and values, a collecting summary could be "You see yourself as a caretaker to others, and being a mother is important to you. You also value reliability and honesty." Collecting summaries can be followed by emptying statements such as "What else?" to ensure that all relevant information has been obtain prior to moving to a different portion of the discussion.

Linking summaries help tie the current conversation back to prior conversation topics. A succinct way to use this sort of summary is to first offer a simple reflection of the current conversation, then link to a prior topic, and provide a reflection of the prior conversation. This can be done organically by statements such as "When you were talking about _____, it was similar to what you'd said earlier about _____" or "How you are feeling now is similar to when you previously experienced _____."

The last category of summaries is transitional summaries. They signal the shift from one topic to another. If collecting summaries can be described as reflect–empty and linking summaries can be defined as reflect–link–reflect, then transitional summaries can be viewed as orient–reflect–empty.

Here is an example of a transitional summary:

1. Orient: "Before we move on to discussing treatment options, would it be okay if I shared my understanding of your struggle with smoking?"
2. Reflect: "You are finding it challenging to stop smoking due to difficulty dealing with cravings for nicotine and with increased stress, and at the same time you are

Motivational Interviewing

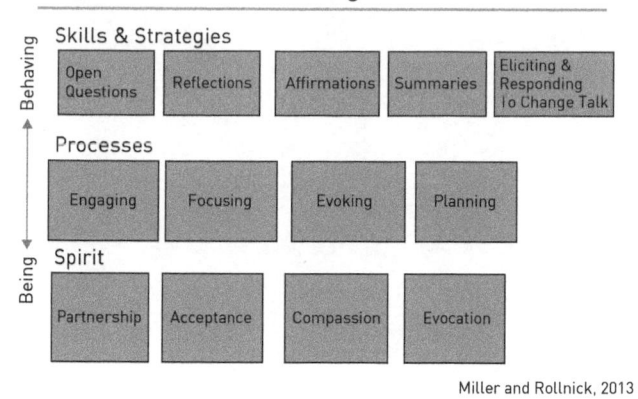

Miller and Rollnick, 2013

FIGURE 2.2. Motivational interviewing: spirit, processes, and skills. From Miller and Rollnick.[2]

motivated to stop smoking due to your asthma, HIV illness, and your concern about your baby's health."

3. Empty: "What other thoughts do you have about your smoking before we discuss a plan?"

The previous reflect transitional summary is an example of a double-sided reflection. Note the use of "and at the same time" rather than "but"; the word "but" tends to negate the clause before it, rather than allowing patients to weight the two different sides of the reflection.

In practicing MI, it is important to keep in mind the four key processes and the core clinical skills and strategies such as reflective listening and eliciting change talk (Figure 2.2). MI facilitates the process of helping patients to explore and resolve their ambivalence about behavior change and address discrepancy between their current behavior and broader life goals and values. Navigating the process of when and how to transition from building motivation to the goal setting and planning phases of behavior change is challenging. The next chapter will build upon the basics by providing strategies to use in clinical practice, helping to guide patients through behavioral change, and managing challenging patient encounters.

REFERENCES

1. Douaihy A, Kelly TM, Gold MA, eds. *Motivational Interviewing: A Guide for Medical Trainees*. New York, NY: Oxford University Press; 2014.
2. Miller WR, Rollnick S. *Motivational Interviewing: Helping People Change*. 3rd ed. New York, NY: Guilford Press; 2013.
3. Moyers TB, Martin T, Christopher PJ, et al. Client language as a mediator of motivational interviewing efficacy: where is the evidence? *Alcohol Clin Exp Res*. 2007;31(10 suppl):40s–47s.
4. Dillard JP, Shen L. On the nature of reactance and its role in persuasive health communication. *Commun Monogr*. 2005;72(2):144–168.
5. Brehm SS, Brehm JW. *Psychological Reactance: A Theory of Freedom and Control*. New York, NY: Academic Press; 1981.

3 Motivational Interviewing Strategies

Priyanka Amin, Antoine Douaihy, and Gordon Liu

A key challenge for the motivational interviewing (MI) practitioner is to facilitate behavior change by accepting and meeting the patient's current level of motivation for change using specific techniques and strategies (Table 3.1). Helping the patients navigate the process of seeing the change as personally important and meaningful and linking it to their core values can enhance motivation for change.

STRATEGIES FOR VARYING LEVELS OF MOTIVATION FOR CHANGE

Lack of motivation for change

Patient: I know that I have HIV, but I feel completely fine, so I haven't been taking HIV medications you prescribed. I don't have any problems with my health, and I don't want to take a medicine that is going to give me side effects.

What looks like 'lack of motivation" is often just ambivalence. The previous statement is from a patient who expresses no intention to take antiretroviral medication. Key strategies to use with patients that express no motivation for behavioral change include listening, building rapport, understanding their perspective, shared agenda setting, open-ended questions, content, feeling, and double-sided reflections. *Expressing curiosity* can facilitate the process of sharing concerns about and reasons for not wanting to take the medications. If patients were confronted with a statement arguing for one side, such as "You need to take the medications anyway," can evoke reactance and defensiveness of the status quo, decreasing the likelihood of change. Such a response could create discord in the relationship, shut the patients down, or make it less likely for them to be honest about medication adherence at subsequent visits. Thus, remaining *empathic, using reflections, and asking evocative questions* move the conversation in a productive way: for example, saying "Since you are feeling healthy, you see no reasons to take the

Table 3.1. Motivational Interviewing Strategies

Motivational Interviewing Strategies	
Ask permission	Would like to know more about antiretroviral therapy (ART)?
Elicit–Provide–Elicit (E-P-E)	What do you know? (E)
	Provide information/offer menu of options (P)
	What do you think?
	What do you make of this information or suggestions? (E)
Importance and confidence rulers	Importance ruler:
	On a scale from 0 to 10 where 10 is the most important and 0 is the least important, what number would you give for how important is to you to (behavior change)? Why did you choose a (current number) instead of a (lower number)? What would you need to do to make it a (higher number)?
	Confidence ruler:
	On a scale of 0 to 10 where 10 is the most confident and 0 is the least confident, what number would you give for how confident you are that you could (behavior change) if you wanted to? Why is it a (current number) instead of a (lower number)? What would you need to do to make it a (higher number)?
Agenda mapping	Ask the patients to set the agenda to focus discussion on what their concerns are. This is also appropriate to do: You shared that you are concerned about your drinking right now and at the same time I am concerned about you have not been taking your ART consistently. Can we discuss this too? what might be the first step to look at both of those goals?

Table 3.1 Continued.

Motivational Interviewing Strategies	
Evoking change talk	What makes you think you need to make (behavior change)?
	What would you like to do differently about your situation?
	What would be the good things about changing (your behavior)?
	What can we work on together to help you change?
	If you were to decide to change, what would you have to do to make this happen?
Normalizing ambivalence	A lot of people struggle to change their behavior.
	Many people are conflicted about making a change.
Shifting focus	Patient: You mentioned that I have to stop drinking, but I don't think I have a drinking problem.
	Practitioner: You are confident that you do not have a drinking problem. Help me understand your drinking pattern.
Agreement with a twist	Patient: Every time I talk with my wife she bugs me about my smoking. Why won't they get off my back and let me be?
	Practitioner: Your wife is worried about your smoking. At the same time it feels like nagging than a way of expressing her concern.
Emphasizing personal choice and control	Patient: You say that I have to take ART and all the other medications every day, but I don't think I can keep up with that.
	Practitioner: Whether you take the medications every day is completely up to you. I definitely would not want you to feel pressured to do something you don't want to do.
Double-sided reflection	Patient: Sometimes I get angry with myself for not coming to the clinic regularly, but I don't have much time because of work and so many responsibilities at home.
	Practitioner: You struggle with keeping up with your appointments at the clinic, at the same time it bothers you when you don't do it as you need to.

medications" argues against change by using an amplified reflection can often lead the patient to reverse course and argue for change. Also consider saying "You are concerned if you take the medications you will be experiencing side effects"; "What is your understanding of what could potentially happen to your HIV illness if you don't take the medications?"; or "What is your understanding of how your medications work?" or elicit permission prior to providing information by asking, "Would it be okay if I share more information on how the medications work and what potential side effects you can experience and how we can address them?" Bringing to the table relevant considerations and consequences of actions and *inviting patients to share* their feelings and thoughts can help guide them from a place of lacking motivation entirely to having more motivation and potentially being willing to establish a shared agenda to continue the conversation and maintain harmony in the therapeutic relationship.

Low Motivation for Change

Patient: I haven't been taking the medications you prescribed, but my partner seems to be getting upset about this. He tries to guilt me into taking them, so I can be healthy for our children. I mean, I want to live a long life and be a healthy mom for them. I don't really like the side effects I get though, and money has been tight lately. I'm not sure what to do, maybe I should take the medications . . .

This statement from a patient illustrates that motivation to engage in a course of action is driven by complicated and competing needs. The emotional intensity of ambivalence is shared by this patient and manifested in change talk and sustain talk, occurring in the same sentence. Resist the righting reflex, meaning taking up the "good" side of the ambivalence, which can backfire and even make the patient unwilling to consider change. The focus here is to explore ambivalence rather than arguing, directing, or "righting." Using double-sided reflections demonstrates both sides of the ambivalence, promotes empathic listening, and recognizes sustain talk and combines it with change statements. Consider the following two reflections to the previous patient statement:

Reflection A: You really want to be healthy for your children and not get into conflicts with your partner, and taking the medication would help you with this goal.

Reflection B: You don't like the side effects of the medication and are worried about financial stressors, and at the same time you really want to be there for your children. You see that taking the medication can help you live longer and healthier.

Patient response to reflection B: Yes I guess I have mixed feelings.

Reflection A does not reflect the internal dilemma that the patient is facing, as it only considers the reasons for change. Reflection B captures the patient's concerns about taking the medications while also reflecting the reasons this patient is considering taking the antiretroviral medications.

The patient has expressed change talk and is cognitively and emotionally considering ramifications of her actions, weighing the pros and cons of current behavior (not taking medications) versus a different behavior (taking medications). She discusses a reason to change: her children. A caveat to this discussion is the issue with perpetuating "sustain talk," which can occur if reflections only convey reasons why someone does not want to consider behavior change. In the previous scenario, it is possible that sustain talk would emerge if only the first clause of reflection B was said. It is best to highlight the "change talk" and end the reflection with it, to help develop discrepancy, which, in turn, can decrease ambivalence regarding behavioral change. Consider the following responses to ambivalence:

Patient: I haven't been taking the medications you prescribed, but my partner seems to be getting upset about this. He tries to guilt me into taking them, so I can be healthy for our children. I mean, I want to live a long life and be a healthy mom for them. I don't really like the side effects I get though, and money has been tight lately. I'm not sure what to do, maybe I should take the medications . . .

Practitioner: Well, you should take the medications. We talked about why you must take them every day, so you need to start taking them as soon as possible. Your medication regimen is way better than it used to be, so you should be happy about that.

Patient: I don't know. I'm not sure I really need them, because I haven't been taking them and feel fine.

Note how the practitioner's response elicited reactance from the patient, who totally dismissed the idea of change. Consider the following reflection, followed by asking permission:

Practitioner: You don't like the side effects of the medication and are worried about financial stressors, and at the same time you really want to be there for your children. You know well that taking the medication can help you live longer and healthier. Would it be okay to discuss ways to help manage the side effects and cost?

Patient: Sure, I'd like that.

This response builds upon the double-sided reflection (reflection B) in the last scenario, while asking permission to discuss ways to manage the patient's concerns. Asking permission allows the patient to retain autonomy in the conversation.

Change talk predicts behavior change and increased commitment strength to the lifestyle change, which in return is correlated to positive clinical outcomes.[1,2] Using strategies to evoke change talk facilitates the direction of the conversation toward a plan of action elicited from the patient:

"If you decided to take your HIV medications, what makes you believe you could follow through with it?"

"What does it mean for you to be a healthy mom?"

"What do you think your partner is concerned about if you don't take the medications?"

"Suppose that you don't take the medications, what is the worst thing that might happen to you?"

"What is the best thing that you could think of that could result from your adherence to medications?"

High Motivation for Change and Moving from Evoking to Planning

Developing and strengthening commitment to change is directly linked to successful behavior change.[3] Following up with the previous vignette, if after a discussion of medication adherence and side effects the patient continued to express more change talk such as reasons for and benefits of change and commitment language to develop a plan to modify adherence to medications behavior, it means that the patient is most likely ready to take the next step in the MI process: committing and panning for change. It is useful to help measure the individual's confidence and motivation for change using a 0 to 10 scale (confidence ruler), with 0 being "not at all confident" or "not at all motivated" and 10 being "extremely confident" or "the most motivated I have ever been." This is a good tool to assess a patient's baseline confidence and motivation and to follow up at subsequent visits or after a discussion using a brief motivational intervention based on MI. If the ratings have shifted, asking follow-up questions such as "What makes you a 6 instead of a 3?" can help the patient think about what internally has led to a change in confidence level. After asking this, the practitioner can follow up by asking "What would need to change before you reach an 8 instead of a 6?" to gain insight into the current barriers the patient is facing. Addressing and encouraging the patient to articulate the reasons for confidence provides an opportunity to envision what success looks like and feels like and what makes it a reasonable outcome.[4,5] Helping patients develop a reasonable plan is crucial at this level of motivation, so that they have a greater chance of sustained behavioral change. Being able to identify signs of readiness to transition to planning is crucial. Some of those signs include an increase in the intensity and frequency of change talk and reduction in sustain talk; small changes in behavior; relief from inner struggles; envisioning the future; and jumping in or "testing the water," meaning that the practitioner could proceed with asking directly about the issue such as "What are your thoughts about discussing possible ways you could consider to move ahead with changing your behavior?" or they could use a less direct way to guide the patient toward the planning process, which involves summarizing the patient's statements related to preparatory and mobilizing change talk and then using an open-ended question about how to proceed.[4] Here's an example:

Patient: I know what I need to do is to take my medications regularly, and I am really committed this time to do it, and I promised my partner to follow through.

Practitioner: You have expressed to me that you have been thinking more seriously about the importance of taking your medications and not missing any doses, and you identified how committed you are to do it because you want to live a healthy life and be there for your children. You have also expressed more confidence that you could follow through with this decision. What do you like to go from here? And what do you believe we could do together that will help you follow through with being adherent and staying adherent to your medications?

As always maintaining the collaborative spirit of MI should guide the discussion with the goal of moving toward planning and implementing change. It is up to the patient to take the leap of faith that is needed to move from thinking and talking about change to making the change.[4,5]

CHANGE IMPLEMENTED

Patient: I've been taking the medications every day.

Practitioner: You have followed through with your decision to take the medications. How have you been doing with that?

Patient: Well, I guess at first it was harder because I forgot to take it some days until my partner reminded me, so I started to use a phone alarm. Since then, I've made it a part of my routine. I feel pretty good!

Practitioner: You feel so encouraged and proud of yourself, and you continue to be motivated to take your medications the way it is prescribed, and you problem-solved to help make it easier to do it.

The patient has now changed his behavior, choosing to take the medications daily. MI can be helpful to continue to explore barriers to sustained behavioral change and ways to address them. It is important to not cheerlead patients by saying "Good job" or "I'm so proud of you!" as they become less likely to disclose if they have had difficulties sustaining change.

MI IN CHALLENGING CLINICAL ENCOUNTERS

Difficult or challenging clinical encounters are very common in clinical practice. The difficulty most likely results from ineffective practitioner–patient communication that, in turn, leads to a breakdown or discord within the relationship.[6] There are challenges that may emerge when attempting to implement MI into clinical practice. To effectively apply MI to help patients build motivation for change, the practitioner must be aware of their own internal experiences and reactions to patients' struggle's and remain open, honest, and nonjudgmental.

As healthcare practitioners, we may be more acutely aware of the risks and long-term sequelae of certain behaviors, such as nonadherence to antiretroviral therapy or engagement in high-risk behaviors such as sharing needles or having unprotected sex. When patients do not follow through with our advice and recommendations, it can engender strong negative feelings toward them such as anger, frustration, sadness, etc., which, in turn, can potentially jeopardize the patient–practitioner relationship and make it less therapeutic. There are several factors that contribute to difficult clinical encounters.[4] The practitioner-specific factors include lack of experience, poor communication skills, desire to be the expert over the patient, practitioner burnout, competing demands and time management issues, clashes with professional identity, cultural gaps, and patient mistrust. The patient-specific factors include psychosocial stressors; mood, anxiety, personality, or substance use disorders; trauma history; nonadherence or poor response to treatment; and previous experiences with ineffective practitioners. Finally, healthcare system characteristics include language and cross-cultural issues, time pressures, competing demands, lack of continuity of care, deficits in interprofessional communication, and reimbursement structures (such as pay for performance). As an egalitarian and collaborative approach opposite to an authoritarian and confrontational style, MI is well-suited to fostering a strong therapeutic relationship that decreases discord and facilitates informed decision-making in challenging clinical encounters. Remaining compassionate and accepting the patient's perspective helps break the unproductive cycle that is associated with challenging encounters. Managing clinical and personal issues through supervision and in vivo coaching, working toward systems changes, and using MI as a therapeutic foundation for all therapeutic encounters can help practitioners address their negative reactions to patients' struggles and complex problems.

The nonadherent patient is an example of a challenging patient. In MI, seeking an understanding of and evoking what is contributing to a patient's nonadherence with treatment is crucial. The approach that commonly emerges here is the righting reflex or desire to fix the problem (discussed earlier). This can translate to lecturing patients on the importance of adherence or asking them why they are not being adherent, which limits patient engagement and unlikely leads to increased adherence. More effective approach such as "What makes it difficult for you to adhere to treatment?" is value-neutral and more likely to elicit challenges and change talk. MI strategies to challenging clinical encounters include exploring the patient's underlying ambivalence and developing discrepancies regarding a patient's current nonadherence and their personal goals and values.[4,5]

DELIVERING BAD NEWS

In caring for people living with HIV, providers will inevitably have to deliver bad news to patients and loved ones. Bad news may be defined as any clinical situation in which "there is either a feeling of no hope, a threat to a person's mental of physical well-being, or a risk of upsetting an established lifestyle."[4p107] Sharing with patients their positive HIV status can be quite challenging. Once the engagement in the encounter starts, MI spirit and skills can be effective in bad news encounters. Using the *elicit–provide–elicit* (E-P-E) framework can be helpful. The initial elicit invites the patients to share their current knowledge and understanding.

> "What do you know about HIV illness and its treatment?"
> "What would it mean to you if your test came back positive for HIV?"

Prior to providing information, explicit permission should be obtained.

> "Would it be okay with you if we discuss the results of your HIV test?"
> "Would you like me to share with you about treatment options?"

After obtaining permission, then the practitioner can provide information in a non-judgmental fashion. Following this should be a second eliciting, this time focusing on the patient's understanding and reactions to the information that has been shared:

> "What are your thoughts about the information I've shared with you?"
> "Now that we have reviewed treatment options, what are your thoughts about you like to do next?"

The latter statement helps bridge into the next part of the discussion, which is generally planning of next steps. Providers may find themselves going back and forth between providing information and eliciting reactions, as clarifications may need to occur.

REFERENCES

1. Martins RK, McNeil DW. Review of motivational interviewing in promoting health behaviors. *Clin Psychol Rev.* 2009;29(4):283–293.
2. Moyers TB, Martin T, Christopher PJ, Tonigan JS. From in-sessions behaviors to drinking outcomes: a causal chain for motivational interviewing. *J Consult Clin Psychol.* 2009;77(6):1113–1124.

3. Miller WR, Rose G. Toward a theory of motivational interviewing. *Am Psychol.* 2009;64(6):527–537.
4. Douaihy A, Kelly TM, Gold MA, eds. *Motivational Interviewing: A Guide for Medical Trainees.* New York, NY: Oxford University Press; 2014.
5. Miller WR, Rollnick S. *Motivational Interviewing: Helping People Change.* 3rd ed. New York, NY: Guilford Press; 2013.
6. Wilson, H. Reflecting on the difficult patient. *N Z Med J.* 2005;118(1212):U1384.

4 Motivational Interviewing and the Continuum of HIV Care in Practice

Shriya Kaneriya, K. Rivet Amico, and Antoine Douaihy

Since the mid-1990s, there has been an 80% decline in the age-adjusted HIV-related mortality rate in the United States.[1] The development of a combination of highly active antiretroviral therapy (HAART), now known simply as antiretroviral therapy (ART), has given people living with HIV (PLWH) the opportunity to control their illness and to live long, healthy, and productive lives. The success in transforming HIV into a chronic manageable condition can be attributed to a coordinated effort across multiple disciplines and stakeholders to advance understanding, options, and interventions in all aspects of the infection, an approach that has since translated into the practical setting for HIV management.[2] Given the broad range of clinical and psychosocial needs of people affected by HIV, a comprehensive interdisciplinary team model has become the standard of care.

THE EVIDENCE BEHIND MOTIVATIONAL INTERVIEWING

Motivational interviewing (MI) is an evidence-based therapeutic counseling style that strengthens practitioner–patient relationships.[3,4] In contrast to more traditional approaches, MI is an egalitarian, person-centered, and empathic way of conversing with patients geared toward resolving ambivalence and enhancing motivation for behavioral change. Instead of instructing patients on what to do, MI focuses on calling out a person's own reasons, resources, and intrinsic motivation for change. The intervention can be blended with other evidence-based clinical practices and approaches to individualize care.

MI is a widely applicable intervention for managing medical conditions in which patient behavior has profound implications on long-term health.[5-7] Over the years, numerous clinical studies have evaluated the effectiveness of MI in comparison with traditional approaches of providing advice for changing behaviors, increasing treatment adherence, and improving health outcomes. These investigations have often focused on the chronic disease management of conditions such as hypertension, diabetes, chronic kidney disease, obstructive sleep apnea, depression, anxiety and substance use disorders.[8] A majority of randomized clinical trials evaluating various parameters demonstrated that MI produces better treatment adherence and health outcomes that have the potential to remain durable over time.[5] Surprisingly, when MI is used in brief, 15-minute clinical encounters, 64% of studies showed a positive patient outcome.[7] Evidence suggests that MI also requires less time than alternative effective strategies to achieve intended results.[3,4] As HIV has now become a chronic, manageable condition, these findings are increasingly pertinent to modern HIV care.

MI is a relatively new intervention in the HIV clinical setting, with its predominant use in the context of disease prevention through reduction of behaviors that risk onward transmission.[9] The EXPLORE study[10] is a randomized control trial investigating behavioral interventions in a large sample of men who had sex with men (MSM) that demonstrated a significant reduction in the rate of HIV infection among those who received MI versus those who received standard counseling sessions. The effectiveness of MI in such interactions may be related to how MI can, over time, strengthen established therapeutic alliances as well as simultaneously address other associated risk factors, such as substance use. Literature pertaining to MI's application to HIV treatment has been evolving rapidly; however, sufficient evidence exists to promote the role of MI in enhancing ART adherence.[11–14] A recent integrative review[15] demonstrated a positive relationship between MI-based interventions and behavioral change, which may lead to improved health outcomes in PLWH. This translates into practical applications of MI as an effective clinical style with individuals who are HIV positive and struggle with adherence, depression, and risky sexual behaviors. There is no concise recommendation on the optimal dose or duration of MI, perhaps because the intervention likely needs to be individually adjusted based on a patient's unique barriers and motivations to change.

There is a well-established evidence for the efficacy of MI in minority populations as well as strong evidence supporting its cross-cultural applicability.[16,17] MI is incredibly versatile in its implementation. Large meta-analyses and systematic reviews have studied whether the profession of an MI interventionist influences behavior change outcomes. Evidence supports the notion that MI is unique in that it can be successfully delivered by a broad scope of healthcare practitioners.[16] This evidence is further reflected in the HIV-specific literature, which demonstrates statistically significant ART adherence outcomes by various practitioners. Interestingly, nurses were found to be the most prevalent MI administrators within the HIV clinical setting.[18] Furthermore, MI is not limited to the traditional in-person format of counseling and can be delivered via telephone-based sessions.[12] This can be especially beneficial for PLWH who may struggle with systemic barriers to care like transportation or the perceived stigma of being seen at a HIV clinic.

THEORETICAL FRAMEWORKS FOR MI IN HIV CARE

Over the past two decades, a number of theoretical models and frameworks have been proposed and used to characterize the determinants of optimal HIV-care outcomes. The information–motivation–behavioral skills (IMB) model[19–22] (Figure 4.1) is frequently used for HIV-related behaviors subsequently articulated to ART adherence specifically. It suggests that three determinants of behavior are needed to engage in

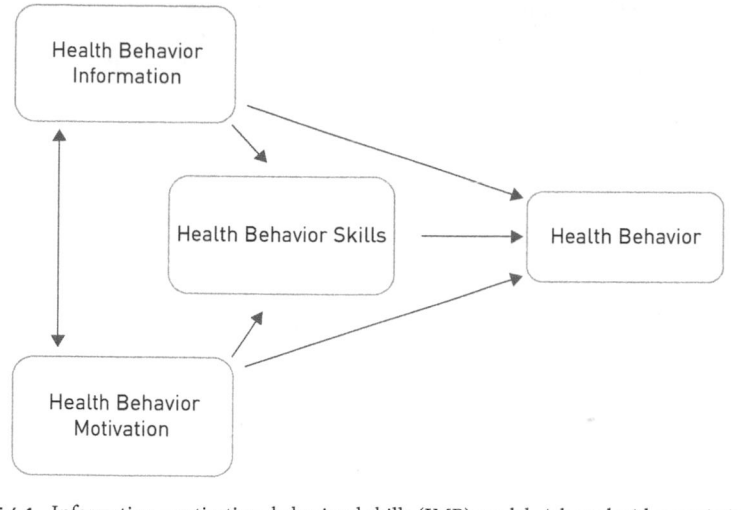

FIGURE 4.1. Information–motivation–behavioral skills (IMB) model. Adapted with permission, Fisher and Fisher, 2000.

a health behavioral change: information, motivation, and behavioral skills. In other words, an individual must be well informed, motivated to act, and possess the appropriate behavioral skills to be effective. Both multivariate correlational and experimental intervention research have supported the model's approach for HIV prevention, ART adherence, and sustained reduction of behaviors that risk onward transmission or infection across a diversity of populations. In this model, the determinant of motivation is divided into two categories: personal motivation, which includes a person's beliefs and attitudes toward a specific health behavior and outcome, and social motivation, which includes the perceived social support or norm for engaging in a specific health behavior. The model was subsequently articulated as a situated model (sIMB)[23] of care initiation and maintenance to engagement in care for chronic medical conditions, where each component of the IMB model is situated within a socio-ecological framework (individual, interpersonal, community, clinic and structural levels of influence). The IMB and sIMB models have used MI to move from models of causes of outcomes to interventions promoting health outcomes. Working with individuals, providers, and communities, clinicians can position information, motivation, and skills as areas for change, while also helping to develop and mobilize mechanisms for change using MI.

Another model well matched to MI principles is the Andersen behavioral model of health service use (ABM)[24-26] (Figure 4.2). Factors affecting retention and adherence to treatment include substance use and psychiatric disorders, social support system, transportation, housing, and healthcare environment factors such as clinic experiences and practitioners' characteristics. ABM has been used to explore these factors affecting healthcare and treatment use among PLWH. MI can be used with this model to engage and retain patients in care and address issues related to substance use and psychiatric illness.

It is not uncommon for any HIV-related practitioner, including physicians, nurses, pharmacists, and case managers, to work with patients adjusting to their diagnosis, treatment regimens, stigma, lifestyle choices, co-morbid illnesses, and the psychosocial implications of what it means for that individual to be HIV-positive. MI is a method for communicating and interacting with individuals, couples, families,

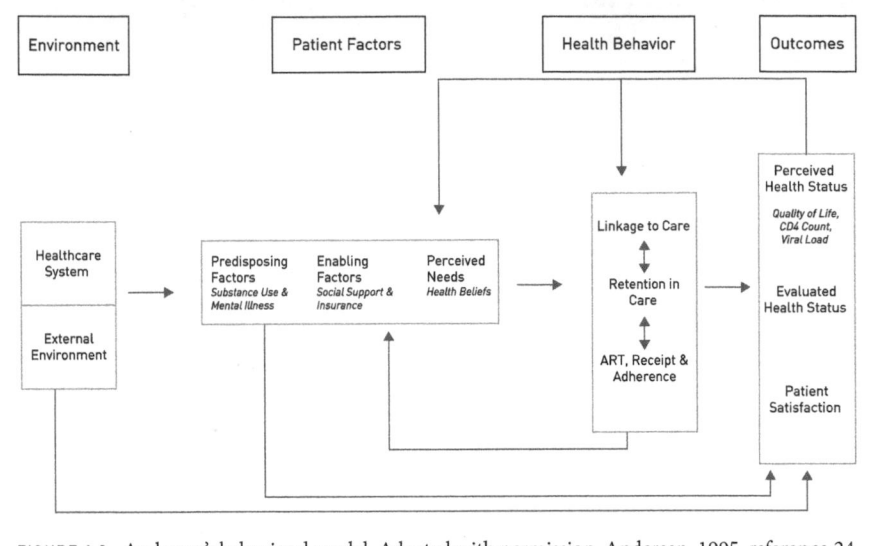

FIGURE 4.2. Andersen's behavioral model. Adapted with permission, Andersen, 1995, reference 24.

and communities. It is important to have a background model or theory for which determinants of health are considered most critical. This centers the MI strategies to guide toward behavioral change following an articulated pathway.

Adopting the MI clinical method in such scenarios can lead to improved risk identification, preventative screening, risk-reduction counseling, positive behavior change, ART adherence, and retention in care (Box 4.1). Many patients feel shame and guilt and are reluctant to share the whole truth regarding intimate struggles and challenges. There may be apprehension in disclosing their HIV status to loved ones due to a fear of disapproval and judgment. MI trains practitioners on how to open up collaborative, empathic, and nonjudgmental clinical encounters. Only when patients are feeling safe to share openly about their struggles can practitioners negotiate and recommend appropriate care plans. ART regimens involve careful daily timing, close follow-up labs, regular clinic appointments, and monitoring of side effects. The pills themselves may carry a sense of stigma for some patients who aren't coping well with their HIV status.

Box 4.1

Positive Behavioral Changes in HIV Care That Can Improve Patient Health Outcomes

- Overall self-management of HIV illness and other comorbid medical conditions
- Taking ART and other medications as prescribed
- Discussing onward transmission (i.e., feelings toward consistent condom use or safer sex practices)
- Reducing problematic substance use, including needle sharing and drug use practices
- Learning healthy coping mechanisms for managing life stressors and societal stigmas
- Keeping regular appointments with healthcare practitioners
- Adopting health promoting lifestyles (nutrition, exercise)

This complexity makes it difficult for many patients to achieve effective adherence. MI can be used to explore patient-specific barriers and develop discrepancy between patient values and choices to assist with behavior modification. Sometimes patients are aware of the risks related to their choices but feel stuck or ambivalent in their present situation. Prefacing conversations with security of safety and confidentiality, supporting autonomy with empathic statements and providing personalized feedback on health risks of specific harmful behaviors (i.e. IV drug use, unprotected sex) can help put patients at ease and build the confidence required to turn burgeoning motivation into action.

MI is an effective and adaptable clinical intervention for integrating the craft and science of medicine to inspire crucial behavioral changes that lead to positive HIV health outcomes. It allows practitioners to focus on specific behaviors, develop insight into factors contributing to patient ambivalence, and have more valuable conversations by meeting patients where they are. The versatility of MI delivery broadens the scope of practice to the variety of healthcare practitioners that make up an interdisciplinary HIV care team. Appropriate and high-quality training in MI is necessary to have a greater influence on patient health outcomes and quality of life.

REFERENCES

1. Centers for Disease Control and Prevention. (2017, June). Fact sheet. HIV Resource Library. https://www.cdc.gov/hiv/pdf/library/factsheets/hiv-viral-hepatitis.pdf. Published June 2017.

2. US Department of Health and Human Services, Health Resources and Services Administration, HIV/AIDS Bureau. Interdisciplinary care teams: a lifeline for people with HIV/AIDS. https://hab.hrsa.gov/sites/default/files/hab/Publications/careactionnewsletter/interdisciplinarycareteamsnewsletter.pdf. Published January 2014.

3. Miller WR, Rollnick S. *Motivational Interviewing: Helping People Change.* 3rd ed. New York, NY: Guilford Press; 2013.

4. Douaihy A, Kelly TM, Gold MA, eds. *Motivational Interviewing: A Guide for Medical Trainees.* New York, NY: Oxford University Press; 2014.

5. Lundhal BW, Kunz C, Brownwell C, et al. A meta-analysis of motivational interviewing: twenty-five years of empirical studies. *Res Soc Work Pract.* 2010;20(2):137–160.

6. Lundahl BW, Moleni T, Burke BL, et al. Motivational interviewing in medical care settings: a systematic review and meta-analysis of randomized controlled trials. *Patient Educ Couns.* 2013;93(2):157–168.

7. Rubak S, Sandbaek A, Lauritzen T, et al. Motivational interviewing: a systematic review and meta-analysis. *Br J Gen Pract.* 2005;55(513):305–312.

8. Westra HA, Aviram A, Doell FK. Extending motivational interviewing to the treatment of major mental health problems: current directions and evidence. *Can J Psychiatry.* 2011;56(11):643–650.

9. Berg RC, Ross MW, Tikkanen R. The effectiveness of MI4MSM: how useful is motivational interviewing as an HIV risk prevention program for men who have sex with men? A systematic review. *AIDS Educ Prev.* 2011;23(6):533–549.

10. Koblin B, Chesney M, Coates T, EXPLORE Study Team. Effects of a behavioural intervention to reduce acquisition of HIV infection among men who have sex with men: the EXPLORE randomized controlled study. *Lancet.* 2004;364 (9428):41–50.

11. Hill S, Kavookjian J. Motivational interviewing as a behavioral intervention to increase HAART adherence in patients who are HIV-positive: a systematic review of the literature. *AIDS Care.* 2012;24(5):583–592.

12. Cook PF, McCabe MM, Emiliozzi S, Pointer L. Telephone nurse counseling improves HIV medication adherence: an effectiveness study. *J Assoc of Nurses AIDS Care.* 2009;20(4):316–325.

13. DiIorio C, McCarty F, Resnicow K, et al. Using motivational interviewing to promote adherence to antiretroviral medications: a randomized controlled study. *AIDS Care.* 2008;20(3):273–283.

14. Maneesriwongul W, Ong-On P, Saengcharnchai P. Effects of motivational interviewing or an educational video on knowledge about HIV/AIDS, health beliefs, and antiretroviral medication adherence among adult Thais with HIV/AIDS. *Pacific Rim Int J Nurs Res.* 2012;16 (2):124–137.

15. Dillard PK, Zuniga JA, Holstad MM. An integrative review of the efficacy of motivational interviewing in HIV management. *Patient Educ Couns.* 2017;100(4):636–646.

16. Hetema J, Steele J, Miller WR. Motivational interviewing. *Annu Rev Clin Psychol.* 2005;1:91–111.

17. Miller WR, Hendrickson SML, Venner K, et al. Cross-cultural training in motivational interviewing. *Journal of Teaching in the Addictions.* 2008;7(1):4–15.

18. Horberg MA, Hurley, LB, Tower WJ, et al. Determination of optimized interdisciplinary care team for maximal antiretroviral therapy adherence. *J Acquir Immune Defic Syndr.* 2012;60(2):183–190.

19. Fisher JD, Fisher WA. Theoretical approaches to individual-level change. In: Peterson J, DiClement R, eds. *HIV Prevention Handbook.* New York, NY: Kluwer Academic/Plenum Press; 2000:3–55.

20. Fisher JD, Fisher WA, Amico KR, Harman JJ. An information–motivation–behavioral skills model of adherence to antiretroviral therapy. *Health Psychol.* 2006;25(4):462–473.

21. Fisher JD, Amico KR, Fisher WA, Harman JJ. The information–motivation–behavioral skills model of antiretroviral adherence and its applications. *Curr HIV/AIDS Rep.* 2008;5(4):193–203.

22. Fisher WA, Fisher JD, Harman JJ. The information-motivation-behavioral skills model: a general social psychological approach to understanding promoting health behavior. In: Suls J, Wallston KA, eds. *Social Psychological Foundation of Health and Illness.* Malden, MA: Blackwell; 2003:82–106.

23. Amico KR. A situated-information motivation behavioral skills model of care initiation and maintenance (sIMB-CIM): an IMB model based approach to understanding and intervening in engagement in care for chronic medical conditions. *J Health Psych.* 2011;16(7):1071–1081.

24. Andersen RM. Revisiting the behavioral model and access to medical care: does it matter? *J Health Soc Behav.* 1995;36(1):1–10.

25. Ulett KB, Willig JH, Lin HY, et al. The therapeutic implications of timely linkage and early retention in HIV care. *AIDS Patient Care STDS.* 2009;23(1):41–49.

26. Holtzman CW, Shea JA, Glanz K, et al. Mapping patient-identified barriers and facilitators to retention in HIV care and antiretroviral therapy adherence to. Andersen's behavioral model. *AIDS Care.* 2015;27(7):817–828.

SECTION II
APPLICATIONS OF MOTIVATIONAL INTERVIEWING INTERVENING IN THE CONTINUUM OF HIV CARE

5 Motivational Interviewing and the Adolescent/Young Adult HIV Care Continuum

Sylvie Naar and Maurice Bulls

Significant progress has been made over the past 30 years in the prevention and treatment of HIV/AIDS. Combination antiretroviral therapy (ART) has transformed infection with HIV from a rapidly debilitating, fatal disease into a chronic disease with high potential for a healthy life for multiple decades.[1,2] Accurate and rapid HIV testing, pre-exposure prophylaxis (PrEP) for individuals at high risk, and viral suppression via ART for individuals who test positive make an AIDS-free generation and the end of the global AIDS epidemic ambitious but achievable national and global goals.[3,4]

Yet despite growing optimism about this potentially achievable outcome, the epidemic remains a major and increasing cause of morbidity and mortality, particularly among adolescents and young adults (hereafter called "youth") and ethnic and racial minorities. Globally, youth living with HIV (YLH) are significantly less likely to receive ART than adults (23% vs. 38%).[3,5–7] In the United States, while the overall HIV incidence from 2003 to 2014 decreased by 25%, among youth aged 13 to 24, it has increased by 43%.[8] Moreover, among youth, new infections have not been evenly distributed. Several minority groups have been overrepresented: almost three fourths of new infections were among men who have sex with men, and over half were among African American youth.[9]

THE YOUTH HIV CONTINUUM OF CARE

The adolescent and young adult HIV treatment cascade is depicted in Figure 5.1 and begins with diagnosis (knowledge of HIV status). Although ~80% of all HIV-positive Americans are aware of their sero-status, only 41% of YLH aged 18 to 24 have this knowledge.[10] Further, knowledge of HIV status among youth does not necessarily result in linkage to care; compared to 75% of adults, more two thirds of YLH are linked to care within 6 to 12 months after diagnosis.[11] Importantly, even linkage to care does not guarantee quality and/or effective care. The physician must initiate ART early, even if there is erratic behavior on the part of the youth, and YLH must recognize that ART

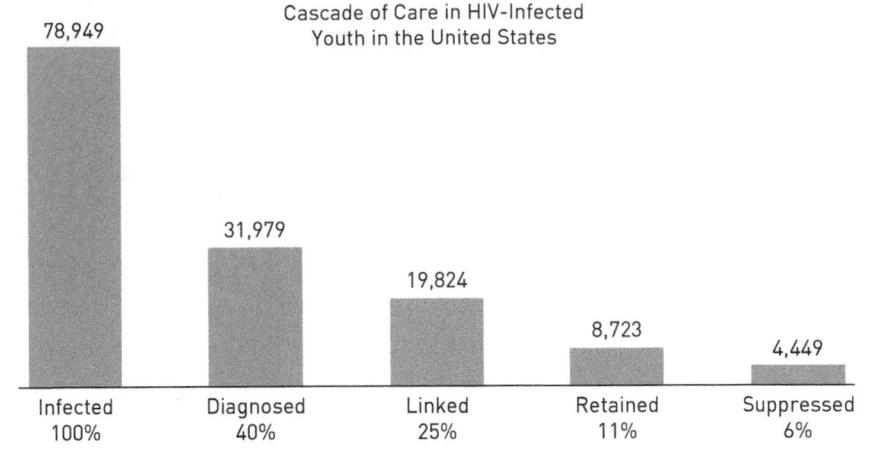

FIGURE 5.1. HIV youth cascade. From Zanoni and Mayer.[11]

is a lifelong commitment and requires a high degree of adherence. Even with appropriate ART initiation and adherence, a small percentage of youth (~10%) are infected with strains of HIV that are already resistant to medications used to treat HIV.[11–13] Further, effectiveness trials report viral suppression rates among YLH receiving ART of >80%, but observational studies (i.e., real-world occurrence) find much lower rates, closer to 50%.[11]

MOTIVATIONAL INTERVIEWING AND THE YOUTH HIV CASCADE

Every step of the HIV treatment cascade, as well as the prevention cascade requires at-risk or YLH to make decisions to engage with the system and/or to modify their behaviors. Motivational interviewing (MI) has been particularly successful in this regard, providing a clear framework for improving patient–provider communication and promoting behavior change using client-centered but goal-oriented methods for enhancing motivation and self-efficacy.[14] High-quality patient–provider relationships consistent with MI are associated with greater likelihood of patients' receiving ART, ART adherence, attending appointments, and having lower viral load.[15–19] MI-consistent approaches produce behavior change and treatment engagement across multiple behaviors, in multiple formats, by multiple disciplines when delivered with adequate fidelity.[20] Fidelity procedures include workshop training by a member of the Motivational Interviewing Network of Training, follow-up coaching with review, and systematic coding of audio-recorded interactions.

MI is central to clinical guidelines for HIV care and HIV risk reduction[16,21–23] and the only intervention approach to demonstrate success across the youth HIV cascade with regard to knowledge of HIV status[16] and retention in care.[18] The Healthy Choices trial demonstrated that four sessions of motivational enhancement therapy (an approach also focused on resolving ambivalence based in MI) compared to standard care significantly improved viral load[24] and reduced risky sex[25] and substance use[26] among youth at highest risk. Healthy Choices is the only meta-analysis currently being tested in an effectiveness implementation trial to improve medication adherence and alcohol use (R01AA022891-01). A pilot trial of Healthy Choices with YLH in Thailand has also shown success,[27,28] and MI is being implemented to improve the HIV youth cascade in the Caribbean.[29]

MI AND ADOLESCENT DEVELOPMENT

Adolescence[30,31] and emerging adulthood is defined as the transitional developmental period between childhood and adulthood, extending from age 12 into the 20s. After infancy, it is the period of the greatest biological, psychological, and social role changes.[32,33] The constant flux of change experienced during this period provides a prime opportunity to intervene and positively alter the trajectory of unhealthy behaviors and poor outcomes.[34] While research on MI has historically focused on adults, two meta-analyses suggest that MI interventions for adolescent substance use retain their effect over time[17] and that the overall effect size of MI was even higher for health behaviors such as diabetes and asthma management.[35]

The normal developmental processes of adolescence regularly affect youth's motivations, decisions, and goals. While the spirit of MI is particularly suited for youth managing identity formation, autonomy pursuits, and impulse control, developmental adaptations may be necessary (see Table 5.1). For example, until patients fully achieve the formal operations stage of cognitive development, abstract thinking may not be fully developed, affecting the patient's ability to think about long-term consequences and answer abstract questions such as "What do you make of that?" In terms of social development, peers become increasingly important and may be a critical source of change talk (CT; discourse suggesting potential reasons for or value of change) and sustain talk (discourse noting reasons not to change). Emotional development of adolescence results in periods of intense emotional lability at times, and making plans for change during these periods may be unwise. In their practical guide, Naar-King and Suarez[36] detail how to use MI with adolescents and young adults.

PATIENT–PROVIDER INTERACTIONS IN YOUTH HIV CLINICS

Literature reviews of MI's mechanisms of effect[36] have concluded that clients' motivational statements about their own desire, ability, reasons, need for or commitment to change (i.e., CT) during MI interactions consistently predict actual client behavior change (see Figure 5.2). Table 5.2 lists examples of CT. In fact, one study of adolescent substance use found that adolescent change talk during sessions predicted marijuana use at 34-month follow-up.[37] A study with adults showed that MI-consistent provider communication was associated with improved HIV medication adherence.[38] However, these studies relied on correlational analyses to identify those provider behaviors most associated with CT; thus, the causal relationship between provider communication and client CT cannot be unequivocally established.

One study of African American adolescents with obesity examined causality in adolescent–provider communication sequences using sequential analysis, a methodology that assesses the probability that CT actually follows specific provider behaviors more likely than chance.[39] The counselor communication behaviors most often leading

Table 5.1. Developmental Implications for MI with Adolescents and Young Adults

Development	Implications for MI
Cognitive development	
Formal operations	Discussions of long-term goals and abstract values may not be as useful for those in earlier stages of development
Information processing	May misinterpret consequences of behaviors and actively seek disconfirming evidence
Social and emotional development	
Identity formation	Allow exploration of self-concept, empathize with ambivalence, and be tolerant of shifts in perspective
Autonomy	Understand that opposition to authority is a normal developmental process
Family	Help family members to reframe adolescent rebellion as normal process of identity formation
Peers	Explore values and stresses associated with peers as possible pros and cons of behavior change
Emotional lability	Careful of making plans for change during period of intense emotion

Type of change talk	Example
Desire	I want to take my meds daily.
Ability	I could make my doctor appointment on my day off.
Reasons	My kids keep me going every day in this battle.
Need	I need to keep viral load low.
Commitment	I'm willing to do anything at this point to make this sick feeling go away.
Takings steps	I am taking my pills every day at 10 am, like clockwork.

to CT included asking open-ended questions to elicit adolescent CT (see Table 5.3) and statements emphasizing adolescents' autonomy (see Table 5.4). Other types of open-ended questions did not significantly elicit CT.

Sequential analysis also identified counselor communication behaviors to avoid because they most often lead to counter-CT or statements against change (e.g., "I don't want to have to come to this clinic for the rest of my life"). These behaviors included open questions to elicit counter-CT, neutral open-ended questions about the target behavior, and reflections of ambivalence (see Table 5.5). Our current analysis of youth–provider interactions in multidisciplinary HIV clinics is showing similar results.

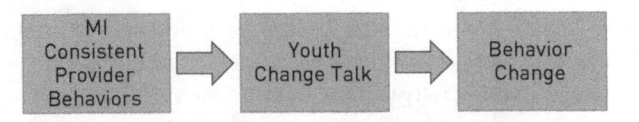

FIGURE 5.2. Mechanism of change in motivational interviewing.

Table 5.2. Youth Change Talk

Type of Change Talk	Evocative Questions
Desire	What are you looking for in this program?
	What is the best thing that would happen if you made a change?
	What do you hope would be better in your life?
Ability	What are some changes that you made before?
	What are some hard things that you have done in the past?
	How likely are you to be able to do this? Why?
Reasons	What are the benefits of making this change?
	What are some reasons you would consider doing this?
Need	What makes this something you need to do?
	How important is it for you do this? Why?
Commitment	What is one thing you can do in the next week?
	How committed are you to making this change? Why?

FUTURE DIRECTIONS

MI was originally developed to build motivation for *initial* change; MI strategies for enacting and maintaining change have begun to be specified in the third edition of the MI text.[40] Once initial motivation for change has been established, it may be time to move to more action-oriented treatments such as cognitive-behavioral therapy (CBT). Thus, incorporating the more action-oriented strategies of CBT may strengthen the behavior changes that MI has helped to initiate. Westra and Arkowitz[41] discuss several ways in which MI can be combined with CBT. First, MI may be delivered as a brief pre-treatment to build motivation for multisession intervention. Second, MI can be used at specific moments during CBT when client discord or ambivalence arises. Third, MI can serve as an integrative framework in which other interventions, such as CBT strategies, could be delivered. Many studies suggest that combining MI with CBT is more effective than usual care in many areas of behavior change such as anxiety,[42] depression

Table 5.3. Open Questions to Elicit Change Talk

Type of Change Talk	Evocative Question
Desire	What are you looking for in this program?
	What is the best thing that would happen if you made a change?
	What do you hope would be better in your life?
Ability	What are some changes that you made before?
	What are some hard things that you have done in the past?
	How likely are you to be able to do this? Why?
Reasons	What are the benefits of making this change?
	What are some reasons you would consider doing this?
Need	Why is this something you need to do?
	How important is it for you do this? Why?
Commitment	What is one thing you can do in the next week?
	How committed are you to making this change? Why?

Table 5.4. Strategies to Emphasize Autonomy

Strategy	Example
Opening statement	Our time today may be different than with other people who have talked to you. I am not telling you what to change or how to change but rather to find out what is going on in your life and support you make the changes that you decide to make.
"You" statements	Your plan is to . . . You said you wanted to . . .
Emphasize choice	Yes, you're right. No one can force you to take medications. You're the one who knows yourself best here. What do you think ought to be on this change plan? What would you like talk about first medications or condoms?
No "should" or "must" statements	You know you should take all your meds. Alternative: Why do you think we recommend taking all your medications? You must follow this treatment plan I give you. You know it's very important Alternative: Why following your plan important you?
Ask for permission	Would it be okay if we discussed some new options to prevent HIV?
Provide a menu of options	What would be the best way to remind yourself of when to take your med—using your phone as an alarm, putting them by your toothbrush, making a schedule and putting it on the refrigerator, or maybe you have something else that may work for you.
Ask for the youth's view	Tell me what you think about those ideas?

Table 5.5. Counselor Behaviors that Elicit Counter-Change Talk

Counselor Behavior to Avoid	Example	Alternative
Open questions to elicit counter-change talk	What makes it so hard for you to come to clinic?	I know it's hard to get here, but what are some of the benefits?
Neutral open questions (questions that do not elicit change talk)	How do you feel about taking medications?	How do you feel about how these medications might help?
Reflections of ambivalence (statements for and against change)	You're not sure about smoking so many times a day, but you feel like you need to smoke marijuana to ease your anxiety.	You're not sure about smoking so many times a day.

with and without comorbid substance use,[43] cocaine use,[44] marijuana use,[45,46] smoking cessation,[47] medication adherence,[48] and weight-related behaviors[49]; however, much less is known about whether either treatment is more effective than a combined treatment approach. While the Healthy Choices trial included some CBT strategies,[50] and an integrated approach has shown some success with adults to improve alcohol use and viral load,[51] MI-CBT interventions have not yet been tested in YLH. A pilot study of MI-CBT for depression in YLH showed promise.[52] Naar and Safren[53] suggest a unified protocol that can be implemented across many target behaviors that utilizes MI to specify the common relational factors of behavioral interventions combined with the common elements of CBT approaches. Future studies are needed to test this unified or transdiagnostic[54,55] approach to target multiple behavior change in YLH.

Despite the success of the Centers for Disease Control program for disseminating evidence-based HIV-related behavioral interventions, a growing body of literature highlights substantial barriers to the effective implementation of these interventions in real-world settings.[56] There have been few studies on implementation of behavioral interventions in HIV care settings,[57] particularly in youth HIV clinics. A new center grant Scale It Up (Naar, S, Parson, JT, Stanton, B, U19HD089875, 2016–2021) in the newly formed Adolescent Trials Network is committed to testing the effectiveness and implementation of MI-based HIV prevention and care interventions to accelerate the translation of research to practice.[58] Future directions include using implementation science to test strategies to promote the delivery of MI with fidelity in real-world settings. Critical questions include how much training is necessary to deliver MI with fidelity, what the newest training models promoted by the Motivational Interviewing Network of Trainers are, how to efficiently and effectively measure fidelity, and what the barriers and facilitators to sustaining MI practice in youth HIV prevention and care contexts are nationally and globally.

For more information about MI training and fidelity measurement, visit www.behaviorchangeconsulting.org.

REFERENCES

1. Kanters S, Mills E, Thorlund K, Bucher H, Ioannidis J. Antiretroviral therapy for initial human immunodeficiency virus/AIDS treatment: critical appraisal of the evidence from over 100 randomized trials and 400 systematic reviews and meta-analyses. *Clin Microbiol Infec.* 2014;20(2):114–122.
2. El-Sadr WM, Holmes CB, Mugyenyi P, et al. Scale-up of HIV treatment through PEPFAR: a historic public health achievement. *J Acquir Immune Defic Syndr.* 2012;60(Suppl 3):S96–S104.
3. Fauci AS, Folkers GK. Toward an AIDS-free generation. *JAMA.* 2012;308(4):343–344.
4. UNAIDS. Fast track: ending the AIDS epidemic by 2030. https://www.unaids.org/en/resources/documents/2014/JC2686_WAD2014report. Published November 18, 2014.
5. Porth T, Suzuki C, Gillespie A, Kasedde S, Idele P. Disparities and trends in AIDS mortality among adolescents living with HIV in low-and middle-income countries. Paper presented at the 20th International AIDS Conference 2014. Melbourne, Australia.
6. Children and AIDS. Children, Adolescents and AIDS. 2014. www.childrenandaids.org
7. United Nations Development Programme. The Millennium Development Goals. http://www.undp.org/content/undp/en/home/sdgoverview/mdg_goals.html.
8. Frieden TR, Foti KE, Mermin J. Applying public health principles to the HIV epidemic: how are we doing? *N Engl J Med.* 2015;373(23):2281–2287.

9. Centers for Disease Control and Prevention. Vital signs: HIV infection, testing, and risk behaviors among youths-United States. *MMWR.* 2012;61(47):971–976.

10. Chen M, Rhodes PH, Hall I, Kilmarx PH, Branson BM, Valleroy LA. Prevalence of undiagnosed HIV infection among persons aged ≥13 years—National HIV Surveillance System, United States, 2005–2008. *MMWR.* 2012;61(2):57–64.

11. Zanoni BC, Mayer KH. The adolescent and young adult HIV cascade of care in the United States: exaggerated health disparities. *AIDS Patient Care STDS.* 2014;28(3):128–135.

12. Gagliardo C, Murray M, Saiman L, Neu N. Initiation of antiretroviral therapy in youth with HIV: a US-based provider survey. *AIDS Patient Care STDS.* 2013;27(9):498–502.

13. Wheeler WH, Ziebell RA, Zabina H, et al. Prevalence of transmitted drug resistance associated mutations and HIV-1 subtypes in new HIV-1 diagnoses, US–2006. *AIDS.* 2010;24(8):1203–1212.

14. Berg RC, Ross MW, Tikkanen R. The effectiveness of MI4MSM: how useful is motivational interviewing as an HIV risk prevention program for men who have sex with men? A systematic review. *AIDS Edu Prev.* 2011;23(6):533–549.

15. Miller WR, Rose GS. Toward a theory of motivational interviewing. *Am Psychol.* 2009;64(6):527–537.

16. Outlaw AY, Naar-King S, Parsons JT, Green-Jones M, Janisse H, Secord E. Using motivational interviewing in HIV field outreach with young African American men who have sex with men: a randomized clinical trial. *Am J Public Health.* 2010;100(Supp 1):S146–S151.

17. Jensen CD, Cushing CC, Aylward BS, Craig JT, Sorell DM, Steele RG. Effectiveness of motivational interviewing interventions for adolescent substance use behavior change: A meta-analytic review. *J Consult Clin Psych.* 2011;79:433–440.

18. Naar-King S, Outlaw A, Green-Jones M, Wright K, Parsons JT. Motivational interviewing by peer outreach workers: a pilot randomized clinical trial to retain adolescents and young adults in HIV care. *AIDS Care.* 2009;21(7):868–873.

19. Parsons JT, Golub SA, Rosof E, Holder C. Motivational interviewing and cognitive-behavioral intervention to improve HIV medication adherence among hazardous drinkers: A randomized controlled trial. *J Acquir Immune Defic Syndr.* 2007;46(4):443–450.

20. Lundahl BW, Kunz C, Brownell C, Tollefson D, Burke BL. A meta-analysis of motivational interviewing: twenty-five years of empirical studies. *Res Social Work Prac.* 2010;20(2):137–160.

21. Bartlett JG, Cheever LW, Johnson MP, Paauw DS. A guide to primary care of people with HIV/AIDS 2004. www.hab.hrsa.gov/tools/primarycareguide. Accessed November 20, 2010.

22. New York State Department of Health. *Substance Use and Dependence Among HIV-Infected Adolescents and Young Adults.* New York, NY: New York State Department of Health; 2009.

23. Centers for Disease Control and Prevention. *Compendium of HIV Prevention Interventions with Evidence of Effectiveness.* Atlanta, GA: Department of Health and Human Services; 2009.

24. Naar-King S, Parsons JT, Murphy DA, Chen X, Harris DR, Belzer ME. Improving health outcomes for youth living with the human immunodeficiency virus: a multisite randomized trial of a motivational intervention targeting multiple risk behaviors. *Arch Pediatr Adolesc Med.* 2009;163(12):1092–1098.

25. Chen X, Murphy DA, Naar-King S, Parsons JT. A clinic-based motivational intervention improves condom use among subgroups of youth living with HIV: a multicenter randomized controlled trial. *J Adolescent Health.* 2011;9(2):193–198.

26. Murphy DA, Chen X, Naar-King S, Parsons JT, Adolescent Trials Network. Alcohol and marijuana use outcomes in the healthy choices motivational interviewing intervention for HIV-positive youth. *AIDS Patient Care STDS*. 2012;26(2):95–100.

27. Rongkavilit C, Naar-King S, Wang B, et al. Motivational interviewing targeting risk behaviors for youth living with HIV in Thailand. *AIDS Behav*. 2013:1–12.

28. Rongkavilit C, Wang B, Naar-King S, et al. Motivational interviewing targeting risky sex in HIV-positive young Thai men who have sex with men. *Arch Sex Behav*. 2014;44(2):1–12.

29. Naar S. Motivational interviewing and the HIV cascade. *International Conference Behavioral Medicine*. Melbourne, Australia; 2016.

30. Park MJ, Paul Mulye T, Adams SH, Brindis CD, Irwin CE. The health status of young adults in the United States. *J Adolescent Health*. 2006;39(3):305–317.

31. Trepper T. Senior editor's comments. In: Worden M, ed. *Adolescents and Their Families: An Introduction to Assessment and Intervention*. New York, NY: Haworth Press; 1991.

32. Rice PF, Dolgin KG. *The Adolescent: Development, Relationships, and Culture*. 12th ed. Boston, MA: Allyn & Bacon; 2008.

33. Arnett JJ. *Emerging Adulthood: The Winding Road from the Late Teens through the Twenties*. New York, NY: Oxford University Press; 2004.

34. Holmbeck GN, Greenley RN, Coakley RM, Greco J, Hagstrom J. Family functioning in children and adolescents with spina bifida: an evidence-based review of research and interventions. *J Dev Behav Pediatr*. 2006;27(3):249–277.

35. Gayes LA, Steele RG. A meta-analysis of motivational interviewing interventions for pediatric health behavior change. *J Consult Clin Psych*. 2014;82(3):521.

36. Apodaca TR, Longabaugh R. Mechanisms of change in motivational interviewing: a review and preliminary evaluation of the evidence. *Addiction*. 2009;104(5):705–715.

37. Walker DD, Stephens R, Roffman R, et al. Randomized controlled trial of motivational enhancement therapy with nontreatment-seeking adolescent cannabis users: a further test of the teen marijuana check-up. *Psychol Addict Behav*. 2011;25(3):474.

38. Thrasher AD, Golin CE, Earp JAL, Tien H, Porter C, Howie L. Motivational interviewing to support antiretroviral therapy adherence: the role of quality counseling. *Patient Educ Couns*. 2006;62(1):64–71.

39. Idalski Carcone A, Naar-King S, Brogan K, et al. Provider communication behaviors that predict motivation to change in African American adolescents with obesity. *J Dev Behav Pediatr*. 2013;34(8):599–608.

40. Miller WR, Rollnick S. *Motivational Interviewing: Helping People Change*: New York, NY: Guilford Press; 2012.

41. Westra HA, Arkowitz H. Introduction. *Cogn Behav Pract*. 2011;18(1):1–4.

42. Westra HA, Arkowitz H, Dozois DJ. Adding a motivational interviewing pretreatment to cognitive behavioral therapy for generalized anxiety disorder: a preliminary randomized controlled trial. *J Anxiety Disord*. 2009;23(8):1106–1117.

43. Riper H, Andersson G, Hunter SB, Wit J, Berking M, Cuijpers P. Treatment of co-morbid alcohol use disorders and depression with cognitive-behavioural therapy and motivational interviewing: a meta-analysis. *Addiction*. 2014;109(3):394–406.

44. McKee SA, Carroll KM, Sinha R, et al. Enhancing brief cognitive-behavioral therapy with motivational enhancement techniques in cocaine users. *Drug Alcohol Depen*. 2007;91(1):97–101.

45. Babor TF. Brief treatments for cannabis dependence: findings from a randomized multisite trial. *J Consult Clin Psych*. 2004;72(3):455–466.

46. Dennis M, Godley SH, Diamond G, et al. The Cannabis Youth Treatment (CYT) study: main findings from two randomized trials. *J Subst Abuse Treat*. 2004;27(3):197–213.

47. Heckman CJ, Egleston BL, Hofmann MT. Efficacy of motivational interviewing for smoking cessation: a systematic review and meta-analysis. *Tob Control.* 2010;19(5):410–416.

48. Spoelstra SL, Schueller M, Hilton M, Ridenour K. Interventions combining motivational interviewing and cognitive behaviour to promote medication adherence: a literature review. *J Clin Nurs.* 2015;24(9–10):1163–1173.

49. Naar-King S, Ellis DA, Idalski Carcone A, et al. Sequential Multiple Assignment Randomized Trial (SMART) to construct weight loss interventions for African American adolescents. *J Clin Child Adolesc.* 2016:45(4):428–441.

50. Naar-King S, Wright K, Parsons J, et al. Healthy Choices: motivational enhancement therapy for health risk behaviors in HIV+ Youth. *Aids Educ Prev.* 2006;18(1):1–11.

51. Parsons JT, Rosof E, Punzalan JC, DiMaria L. Integration of motivational interviewing and cognitive behavioral therapy to improve HIV medication adherence and reduce substance use among HIV-positive men and women: results of a pilot project. *AIDS Patient Care STDS.* 2005;19(1):31–39.

52. Kennard BD, Brown LT, Hawkins L, et al. Development and implementation of health and wellness CBT for individuals with depression and HIV. *Cogn Behav Pract.* 2014;21(2):237–246.

53. Naar S, Safren S. *Motivational Interviewing and CBT.* New York, NY: Guildford Press; 2017.

54. Barlow DH, Allen LB, Choate ML. Toward a unified treatment for emotional disorders. *Behav Ther.* 2004;35(2):205–230.

55. Newby JM, McKinnon A, Kuyken W, Gilbody S, Dalgleish T. Systematic review and meta-analysis of transdiagnostic psychological treatments for anxiety and depressive disorders in adulthood. *Clin Psychol Rev.* 2015;40:91–110.

56. Norton WE, Amico KR, Cornman DH, Fisher WA, Fisher JD. An agenda for advancing the science of implementation of evidence-based HIV prevention interventions. *AIDS Behav.* 2009;13(3):424–429.

57. Schackman BR. Implementation science for the prevention and treatment of HIV/AIDS. *J Acquir Immune Defic Syndr.* 2010;55(Supp 1):S27–S31.

58. National Institute of Health. Program Announcement (PAR-13-055). *Dissemination and Implementation Research in Health (R01).* http://grants.nih.gov/grants/guide/pa-files/PAR-13-055.html. Published January 9, 2013.

6 An Example Program of Motivational Interviewing–Informed Linkage to HIV Care

The Linkage to Care Demonstration Study

Risa Flynn and Robert Bolan

Linkage to HIV care once a patient is diagnosed positive is a critical entry step into the continuum of HIV care.[1] To provide an example of how strategies and approaches based on motivational interviewing (MI) can facilitate linkage in real-world settings, we provide an overview of one program that developed organically as our center sought to better engage clinics from testing to care initiation. Aspects of our program that emphasize the MI Spirit and strategies, as well as lessons learned are provided.

BACKGROUND

In 2011, a consortium of community-based organizations and academic institutions in collaboration with the Los Angeles County Department of Public Health was awarded a grant by the California HIV Research Program to study the HIV continuum of care. The proposal, Pre-Exposure Prophylaxis and Testing, Linkage, Plus for HIV Prevention (PATH), encompassed biomedical and behavioral interventions targeted to increasing testing among high-risk HIV-negative populations, pre-exposure prophylaxis (PrEP) implementation in a community-based clinic, improving linkage to and retention in HIV care, and re-engaging out-of-care patients. The linkage to care (LTC) demonstration project was entitled Linkage to Care: An Evaluation and Examination of a Program to Link Newly Infected HIV Patients to Primary HIV Care. This practice-based intervention, designed to facilitate emotional and cognitive responses for rapid linkage to HIV care, was implemented at the Los Angeles LGBT Center's Sexual Health and Education Program (SHEP), one of the largest HIV testing and care facilities in Los Angeles County. Co-located with an HIV clinic, pharmacy, mental health services, and substance use treatment services, among other medical and social services, there were 16,000 HIV testing visits and 11,000 unique clients in 2013, the first year of the project. The positivity rate was 2.89%, with 257 acute HIV diagnoses in that year, and 3,000 HIV patients in care.

The first analysis of SHEP LTC data in 2009 reported a 46% linkage rate,[2] defined as a provider visit within 6 months of diagnosis. Structural interventions in 2010, including additional staff and protected appointment slots for new HIV diagnoses, resulted in an increased linkage rate of 69%. In 2012, a dedicated LTC specialist (LTC-S) was hired and developed a client-centered approach to LTC, modeled upon the primary principles of MI. This individual was a licensed clinical social worker who had long been conducting HIV disclosures in SHEP prior to this project.

The demonstration project, conducted between March 2014 through September 2015, was designed to systematically evaluate LTC intervention and its outcomes. The primary outcome was LTC within 3 months of diagnosis, and secondary outcomes included retention in care and viral suppression. The investigators sought to identify factors positively and negatively associated with rapid LTC and to administer a cognitive/affective survey within 2 weeks of diagnosis to evaluate barriers and facilitators to linkage and retention. The overall goal was to develop a best practices, replicable protocol for LTC in other community settings. Of 389 newly HIV-diagnosed persons who were eligible at baseline (over 18 years of age, newly diagnosed within 3 weeks prior to enrollment, able to complete a survey in English or Spanish), 118 were enrolled. Thirty-nine eligible individuals (10%) were judged by the LTC-S to be too emotionally fragile upon learning their diagnosis to invite them to participate in a research demonstration project. Of the enrolled participants, 111 (94.1%) attended their first medical visit within 3 months of diagnosis.[3]

APPLICATION OF MI TO LINKAGE TO CARE INTERVENTION

The LTC intervention is rooted in Antiretroviral Treatment Access Study (ARTAS), the strengths-based, brief case management intervention that incorporates motivational strengths-based case management techniques to link recently diagnosed HIV-infected persons to care.[4] Viewing linkage from the socio-ecological perspective, ARTAS emphasizes the nonlinear array of individual, relationship, community, and healthcare system factors at play in the process of linkage.[5]

MI allows clients the freedom to explore their concerns and react to a new HIV diagnosis. The individually tailored methods facilitate organic development of goals and a plan that is reflective of each client's unique resources and readiness. Other approaches based upon MI[6] have established the primacy of self-efficacy and autonomy as components of the brief interventions that most consistently led to successful linkage.

INTERVENTION DESCRIPTION

The LTC-S intervention is organized into three phases. Phase 1 consists of client centered, resiliency-based counseling and support, provided at or soon after diagnosis, which results in actionable goals. The LTC-S begins by allowing the client to react to the diagnosis and discuss their immediate concerns. The focus is on developing rapport and meeting the client's response and ambivalence around their diagnosis without judgment or comment on its apparent efficacy.

The main objectives of Phase 1 are to establish a support plan and a linkage plan, by helping the client identify their own internal strengths and abilities. The counselor assesses individual sources of support, gauges the individual's readiness, provides referrals (e.g., counseling, substance use recovery, group therapy, etc.) and schedules appointments (e.g., financial screening, entry visit) as necessary and appropriate. As needs emerge, potential strategies and related self-care goals are discussed. To develop the linkage plan, the counselor attempts to normalize strong emotional reactions to the HIV diagnosis and describe the desired process for adjusting, navigating, and entering HIV care. The purpose is to guide clients toward a view that LTC is a positive, adaptive response. The collaborative establishment of support and linkage plans encourages clients to feel both autonomous and supported, promoting a sense of personal control over their self-care decisions.

Phase 2 provides immediate follow-up and support as needed between the time of diagnosis and LTC. The counselor encourages the perception of a responsive care system by demonstrating flexibility and availability. During this time before linkage, the counselor conducts as many additional meetings, phone calls, text messages, emails, or other communications as individual need dictates. The counselor affirms and supports decisions that have already been made. The counselor helps to identify and discuss ways to overcome personal or system-based barriers to care. They use the interactions to help clients feel supported as they work through the initial crisis and the process of disclosing to friends, partners, and loved ones. This continued emphasis on personal and social connectedness helps fight against the propensity for isolation and helps clients' growing positive regard for the LTC-S begin to generalize to the clinic as a whole and the entire care team. The LTC-S also uses these conversations to help clients develop or reinforce concrete skills to facilitate the process of entering care.

Phase 3 consists of increasing or decreasing intensity of outreach, based upon monitored linkage status and the client's readiness to engage in care. For those who are ready to link immediately or very soon after diagnosis, the counselor assists with healthcare system navigation, referrals, and scheduling and tapers contact as the patient transitions to their care team. For individuals who are interested in linking to care but may not be ready, the counselor identifies ways to strengthen the client's familiarity with the care team. If appointments are missed, the counselor begins more intensified contact to identify challenges and specific barriers to care. The counselor strategizes with the patient, addressing issues they feel are more pressing than HIV care and rescheduling appointments as needed. For patients who rebuff all attempts at contact, the LTC-S makes periodic efforts to re-engage them until they link or ask the LTC-S to stop reaching out. Using a nonjudgmental approach and remaining supportive to continue building trust and rapport, the LTC-S is able to identify windows of opportunity for education and connection, increasing the chances of interacting at a moment when the client has a sense of readiness to engage in care.

PRIMARY MI TECHNIQUES EMPLOYED

This intervention has multiple characteristics that reflect evidence-based MI principles. The primary tenet of this LTC approach is a client-centered counseling style.

In contrast with a problem-solving, instructive style, MI promotes autonomy so that clients can tap into their own strength and competence to make changes. Beginning with the premise that clients have the power, confidence, and resiliency to make healthy choices enhances their natural, inherent self-motivation toward health and well-being.

Also, distinctly different from an authoritative strategy, MI providers focus on a style that builds collaboration and rapport, rather than an expert–recipient relationship. Instead of providing information, specific strategies, and techniques, the provider asks open-ended questions, reflects the client's observations, and seeks the client's opinion about their choices. In an atmosphere of acceptance and compassion, the client can look inward to identify internal resources and skills they can call upon to make change.

Practitioners of MI have been described as having a unique "way of being," encompassing more than having mastered a set of counseling techniques. The provider's interpersonal skills as they engender a personal, individualized relationship are key. A qualitative evaluation of Wisconsin's HIV LTC intervention, targeted to African American MSM, identified the client's relationships with the LTC-S as a "major, unifying theme. . . . Comfortable and close relationships with Specialists served as motivation to adhere to medical care, mitigated negative feelings associated with HIV-related stigma, and resulted in increased comfort with medical care and positive health outcomes including engagement in care and undetectable viral load."

LESSONS LEARNED

Facing an HIV diagnosis can be a staggering, overwhelming, life-changing process. Even for patients who aren't surprised by the news, the need to begin navigating the complexities of HIV care can generate tremendous ambivalence. The PATH LTC intervention at the Los Angeles LGBT Center's SHEP demonstrated that one key to a sustained, high rate of linkage to HIV care is a well-trained, dedicated, thoughtful clinician utilizing the tools of MI. A provider who brings respect, patience, and a firm

---

MI in the Delivery of HIV-Positive Test

Important features of MI to incorporate in delivery of HIV-positive test result and LTC are as follows.
- Anyone working with delivering HIV diagnoses should be prepared to engage clients in discussion about reactions to the result and the immediate next steps and provide a safe space for diverse, potentially intense, reactions, knowing MI strategies and concepts can help with this.
- Embrace ambivalence when it comes to linking to care or other aspects of learning one's HIV status (e.g., partner notification, disclosure to important others) is preferable to confronting it.
- Meet fear with compassion rather than shutting down conversations about anxiety and sorrow.
- Correct misinformation with education using elicit–provide–elicit.
- Ask permission before offering suggestions or ideas for moving forward.
- Provide affirmation.
- Allow for uncertainty and careful decision making.

belief in clients' ability to find their way through to making healthy change, can significantly impact linkage to HIV care.

REFERENCES

1. Mugavero MJ, Amico KR, Horn T, Thompson MA. The state of engagement in HIV care in the United States: from cascade to continuum to control. *Clin Infect Dis.* 2013;57(8):1164–1171.
2. Bolan R, Beymer M, Gonzalez R, Flynn R. Experience at a community-based LGBT Organization with integrated HIV/STI testing and HIV care. Paper presented at: 6th IAS Conference on HIV Pathogenesis Treatment and Prevention July 2011, Rome, Italy.
3. Bendetson J, Dierst-Davies R, Flynn R, et al. Evaluation of a client-centered linkage intervention for patients newly diagnosed with HIV at an urban United States LGBT center: the linkage to care specialist project. *AIDS Patient Care STDS.* 2017;31(7):283–289.
4. Gardner LI, Metsch LR, Anderson-Mahoney P, et al. Efficacy of a brief case management intervention to link recently diagnosed HIV-infected persons to care. *AIDS.* 2005;19(4):423–431.
5. Broaddus MR, Hanna CR, Schumann C, Meier A. "She makes me feel that I'm not alone": Linkage to care specialists provide social support to people living with HIV. *AIDS Care.* 2015;27(9):1104–1107.
6. Hightow-Weidman LB, Jones K, Wohl AR, et al. Early linkage and retention in care: findings from the outreach, linkage, and retention in care initiative among young men of color who have sex with men. *AIDS Patient Care STDS.* 2011;25(Suppl 1):S31–S38.

7 Incorporating Motivational Interviewing into Interventions to Address Adherence to Antiretroviral Therapy

Carol Golin, Breana Uhrig Castonguay,
Steve Bradley-Bull, and
Catherine Grodensky

RATIONALE AND EVIDENCE FOR THE USE OF MOTIVATIONAL INTERVIEWING TO ADDRESS ANTIRETROVIRAL ADHERENCE

Overview of Antiretroviral Adherence Importance and Challenges

Highly active antiretroviral therapy (HAART), which became widely available in the mid-1990s, has led to a striking decrease in both morbidity and mortality related to HIV/AIDS infection.[1-4] It is now widely recognized that individuals who maintain an undetectable plasma HIV-1 RNA (viral load) can live a healthy, nearly normal lifespan and have markedly reduced risk of transmitting HIV to other individuals.[5-9] Research indicates that adherence to HAART is the strongest predictor of viral suppression, resistance, disease progression, and death.[4,10,11] Assisting patients living with HIV to maintain excellent antiretroviral adherence has become a cornerstone of HIV treatment recommendations. In addition, theoretically, achieving timely diagnosis, linkage, and retention in care and high levels of adherence among all HIV-infected persons could substantially reduce—if not eliminate—the HIV epidemic.[12-14]

Early on, antiretroviral therapy (ART) regimens were highly complex as they required multiple daily doses of numerous medications with severe side effects and also required near-perfect adherence to stave off the development of virologic resistance. Although current medication regimens are simpler, more tolerable, more forgiving, and recognized as critical to successful HIV treatment, the lifelong nature and associated stigma of ART cause some patients to continue to face challenges with consistent adherence. Multiple factors have been shown to influence medication adherence for people living with HIV (PLWH), including, but not limited to, the regimen's fit with daily lifestyle and the individual's perceived HIV-related stigma, literacy level, relationship with their HIV care provider, mental health, substance use, and motivation and self-efficacy to adhere.[4,15-34]

As adherence is a complex behavior with multiple determinants that vary from person to person,[15,35] interventions to address adherence must be individually tailored to address barriers and facilitators. Given the extensive literature demonstrating that numerous barriers to antiretroviral adherence occur at multiple levels of a socioecological framework, comprehensive patient-centered interventions are most likely to be effective. The individually tailored nature of motivational interviewing (MI), an effective theory-based, client-centered counseling approach[36-42] makes it a promising strategy for addressing the complex, multidimensional features of HAART adherence.[43-47]

Existing Evidence for the Efficacy and Effectiveness of Motivational Interviewing to Address Antiretroviral Adherence

In this section, we present the findings of a narrative literature review of studies that used MI-based interventions to improve antiretroviral adherence.[8,9,12-14,48] We focused our literature search on MI intervention studies published within the past 15 years that used a randomized controlled trial (RCT) study design. We then hand-searched study references for other MI-based interventions not identified in our initial search. We identified 5 study characteristics and 7 intervention characteristics to report across studies. For study characteristics, we reported type of RCT, country, setting (academic, clinical, or community), sample size, and study population (see Table 7.1). For MI intervention characteristics, we reported who delivered the MI intervention (and how they were trained); what type of MI program was administered, including mode of delivery and use of supplemental materials; how many sessions (i.e., frequency of the MI program); how MI fidelity was assessed—meaning how the program was evaluated; and, lastly, how medication adherence was measured (see Table 7.1).

Our narrative review revealed effective MI programs are delivered by MI-trained staff and place emphasis on measuring MI program fidelity. MI program fidelity refers to how well the program and its counselors follow MI principles. In our review, nurses delivered most of the MI programs and had received between 1 and 5 days of dedicated MI training by MI trainers, including those who were members of the Motivational Interviewing Network of Trainers (MINT). In addition to these initial trainings, effective studies reported offering MI booster sessions and hosting biweekly team meetings to review challenging cases and conduct role-play exercises. A 2009 systematic review of MI training[61] supports our findings regarding the importance of MI-educated trainers ongoing booster sessions *and* introduces the need for training programs to cover the fundamental principles and skills of MI developed by Miller, Rollnick, and Moyers.[62] To measure MI program fidelity, principal investigators either supervised or listened to audiotaped recordings of a sampling of MI sessions. All effective studies used an independent coder to assess MI quality and most reported using the standardized Motivational Interviewing Treatment Integrity (MITI) coding system. Madson and colleagues[63] evaluated the MITI as a measure for MI fidelity and reported other MI fidelity measures, such as the Motivational Interviewing Skill Code

Table 7.1. Characteristics of Studies That Used MI-Based Interventions to Improve Antiretroviral Adherence

	AUTHOR (YEAR)	SAMPLE SIZE (COUNTRY)	POPULATION (AGES)	SETTING	PROVIDER (AMOUNT OF TRAINING)	MI DELIVERY	ADHERENCE MEASURE	MI FIDELITY MEASURE	FINDINGS
2 ARM RCTs	Dilorio[44] (2008)	247 (USA)	HIV		(24 hours)	3, 1, 4, or			+ −
	Pradier[49] (2003)	202 (France)	HIV		(5 days)	6, 6			+
	Golin[50] (2006)	141 (USA)	HIV		M (24 hours)	3, 2			+ −
	Samet[51] (2005)	151 (USA)	HIV		(not reported)	3, 1			−
	Parsons[52] (2007)	143 (USA)	HIV		M (not reported)	3, 8		MITI	+ −
	Holstad[53] (2011)	203 (USA)	HIV		(24 hours)	2, 8			+ −
	Konkle-Parker[54] (2011)	73 (USA)	HIV		(18 hours)	6, 2, 6		MITI	+ −
	Naar-King[55] (2013)	76 (USA)	HIV (16–24)		N/A	2		N/A	+
	Jones[56] (2016)	120 (Argentina)	HIV		(2 sessions)	1, 4		NR	+ −
3 ARM RCTs	Goggin[57] (2013)	204 (USA)	HIV		(not reported)	6, 6, 4			−
COHORT	Cook[58] (2009)	98 (USA)	HIV		(8 hours)	6, 1–4			+
FEASABILITY & QUALITATIVE	Markham[59] (2009)	32 (USA)	HIV (13–24)		N/A	1		N/A	+
	Outlaw[60] (2014)	10 (USA)	HIV (18–24)		N/A	1, 2	N/A	N/A	N/A

KEY

POPULATION
- History of Alcoholism
- HIV Positive
- Women
- Youth

SETTING
- Academic/Research Hospital or Center
- Clinic(s)
- Community Organization
- NIH Adolescent Trials Network Sites

PROVIDER & TRAINING
- Counselor
- Health Educator
- MINT Standardized
- Multiple Providers
- Nurse or Nurse Practitioner

MI DELIVERY
- Computer Sessions
- Group Sessions
- Home Visits
- In Person Sessions
- Months of MI Intervention
- Supplemental Materials
- Telephone Sessions

ADHERENCE MEASURE
- Electronic Pill Cap
- Pill Count
- Rx Refill Rate
- Self Reporting
- N/A   Not Applicable
- NR   Not Reported

FIDELITY MEASURE
- Review of Written Materials
- Review of A/V Materials
- Personal Observation
- MITI   MITI Coding

FINDINGS
- −   No Significant Results
- +   Significant Results

(MISC), in a 2006 systematic review. They concluded the importance of choosing the appropriate measure for one's sample to ensure one's program follows the original intent of MI.

In addition to the importance of MI-trained staff and measuring program fidelity, successful MI-based interventions provided supplemental materials throughout the MI intervention. In our review, 6 out of 10 interventions that reported some statistically significant results also reported using supplemental materials. Supplemental materials varied across studies and included booster letters mailed after each MI visit,[50] videos of peers discussing how they addressed barriers to purse medication adherence, small-sized inspirational calendars, and wallet-sized cards to facilitate adherence for hazardous drinkers.[52] Authors report that supplemental materials help reinforce intervention components. For example, while not formally tested, there was noted to be a peak (see Figure 7.1[50]) in electronically measured adherence among the Participating and Communicating Together (PACT) intervention participants[50] after they received the MI session and mailed the booster letter (see Figure 7.2 for an example of a booster letter template), which is consistent with prior research demonstrating decays in adherence over time without an intervention.[64] To that end, the timing of supplemental materials in the MI program is important. For Parsons et al.,[52] the MI intervention at 3 months was statistically effective but did not sustain effectiveness at 6 months. Authors reported this may have been because all 8 sessions were completed within 3 months of the baseline visit and participants were no longer receiving the intervention or supplemental materials. These findings support the importance of providing continuous, ongoing MI intervention supplemental materials to maintain behavior change.

Despite the previous components of successful MI programs, there is limited and inconsistent evidence of the effectiveness of MI interventions for ART adherence and

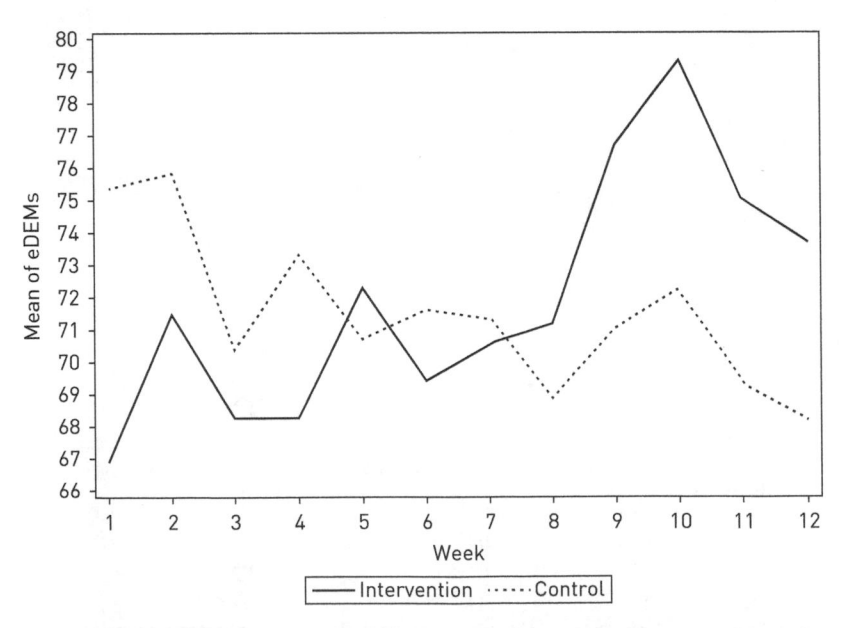

FIGURE 7.1. Results from the Participating and Communicating Together (PACT) randomized controlled trial: comparison of PACT MI-based intervention and control group regarding electronically monitored ART adherence over 12 weeks.[50] eDEMs = Electronic Drug Event Monitoring System.

<<Month date, Year>>

Dear <<patient name>>,

Thank you again for meeting with me the other day. I enjoyed spending time with you and listening to what was on your mind. Like I said when we met, this letter is to remind you of what we talked about.

As you may remember, we talked about <<INSERT SELECTED TOPIC, SUCH AS getting all of the information that you want about your health from your doctor>>.

Some things you brought up were:

NOTE: <<INSERT SPECIFIC SALIENT ISSUES DISCUSSED, SUCH AS:

   o Paying for and taking your medicines.

   o That you're getting good care and good results and you want to kept this up.

   o That recently, some of the assistance you've been getting for your medicines has gotten cut.

   o But, you know of resources that may be available to you through the VA, you've already sought help from the hospital financial counselors, and you know that these might help you continue to pay for your pills.

   o Some things you're planning on doing are setting up an appointment with the Clinic social worker, talking with the hospital financial counselors, and looking into VA benefits >>

With this letter I have included another copy of a list of different ideas that some people have found helpful. I look forward to seeing you again in the <<INSERT CLINIC. on <<INSERT DAY, DATE>> at <<INSERT TIME>> and hearing about how things have been going for you. In the meantime, if you have any questions or need to change your appointment, please call me at (XXX) XXX-XXXX.

Best wishes,

<<*Counselor Sign Here*>>

<<Insert Counselor Name>>

FIGURE 7.2. Sample booster letter template from the PACT trial. RCT = randomized controlled trials. NIH = National Institutes of Health. MINT = Motivational Interviewing Network of Trainers. MI = motivational interviewing. A/V = audio/visual.

a need for more high-quality studies that address key limitations. In a 2012 review of ART interventions using MI by Hill et al.,[65] 3 out of 5 studies report statistically significant adherence changes. However, authors reported methodological concerns such as small sample sizes, intervention participants not receiving the full MI program, the short duration of MI programs, and the need for a universally accepted measure for ART adherence.

Similar to the Hill et al.[65] review, our narrative review showed studies reported null or varied findings (see Table 7.1) due to small sample sizes, duration of MI programs, and inconsistent ART adherence measures. Additionally, measures of adherence varied significantly across studies with most using self-report measures only and few using ART adherence measures that are more objective and shown to be more accurate and reliable, such as Medication Event Monitoring System (MEMS)

> **Box. 7.1**
>
> Main Takeaways from the Narrative Literature Review
>
> - **Training those who deliver your MI intervention:** Choose a program that follows the principles of MI developed by Miller and Rollnick; use a trainer who is a member of MINT; provide booster sessions throughout your MI program.
> - **Measuring MI fidelity:** Choose an MI fidelity measure such as MISC or MITI to ensure you are following MI principals in your program.
> - **Program length:** Consider MI interventions of at least 6 months in duration.
> - **ART adherence measures:** In addition to self-report measures, when possible, choose validated and reliable objective adherence measures, such as pill counts, pharmacy refill records, electronic monitors, or medication levels in hair.

caps, pill counts, or pharmacy refill data. Box 7.1 provides a recap of the main takeaway points from this narrative literature review.

LESSONS LEARNED IN DEVELOPING AND IMPLEMENTING MOTIVATIONAL INTERVIEWING-BASED ANTIRETROVIRAL ADHERENCE INTERVENTIONS

At our institution, we have developed several MI interventions for PLWH,[43,46,50,66–68] including those designed to improve antiretroviral adherence. These MI interventions were grounded in 2 leading health behavior theories: social cognitive theory[69] and the information-motivation-behavioral skills model.[70] Social cognitive theory posits that whether an individual successfully carries out and maintains a learned behavior, like medication-taking, is determined by the interactions between the individual's beliefs about their self-efficacy to perform the behavior, experienced responses to the behavior, and environmental factors.[69] For example, individuals with high self-efficacy, or confidence in their ability to do the behavior, are theoretically more likely to adopt adherence behaviors. The information-motivation-behavioral model asserts that HIV-related information, motivation, and behavioral skills, including medication-taking proficiency,[71] drive antiretroviral adherence.[70,72,73] Based on these concepts and information from quantitative and qualitative research of barriers to antiretroviral adherence, we first designed PACT[50] which was tested in a randomized trial and then refined and adapted for several other settings, including in the imPACT intervention among HIV-infected released prisoners. These interventions included between 2 and 8 MI sessions, delivered biweekly or monthly, in which a trained MI counselor used an MI guide to facilitate the client through a series of nonjudgmental counseling steps that include rapport building, values clarification, selection of an adherence-related topic to address, assessing motivation and self-efficacy to address it, identifying barriers to adherence, developing potential strategies to overcome barriers, and setting goals.

To ensure that MI is implemented with fidelity in these projects and thereby improve our ability to evaluate its effect on medication adherence, our team has created an ongoing program focused on MI and MI-based adherence support implementation that involves training, supervision/coaching boosters, and coding. In the following section, we describe several components of preparation, skill-building, ongoing support, and evaluation we use for MI-based research projects to increase intervention fidelity and enhance MI quality.

SPECIFIC TIPS, TAILORING, AND MODIFICATIONS RELATED TO USING MI FOR MEDICATION AND ART ADHERENCE

Training

MI interventionists in research and clinical settings vary in the training they receive, in part because there is no governing body or licensure for the technique. MINT is an international organization of trainers committed to improving the experience of clients in exploring behavior change. MINT offers a 3- or 4-day training of new trainers (TNT) each year. Once trained, trainers can offer trainings to others seeking to develop or refine behavior change programs tailored to the needs and interests of particular populations. After an individual completes a MINT-sponsored TNT, they are eligible to become a member of the MINT. Two members of our team have been trained through this organization. It should be noted that in many settings people not trained through MINT offer MI training. Based on training through MINT, supplemental resources about MI,[74,75] and experiences training providers and providing MI counseling first-hand in a variety of settings, we have developed a basic training model that we use in our studies focused on the principles and skills of MI. Aspects of the training receiving particular attention included the following.

- *Background information about the target behavior (ART adherence).* Although the primary function of MI is not education, often factual information about the benefits of the target behavior are requested by the client and can be instrumental in enhancing their motivation and self-efficacy. For that reason, our trainings for ART adherence interventions include didactic and interactive modules to increase counselors' understanding of ART medication adherence, the prevalence of nonadherence, techniques for measuring adherence, and factors affecting adherence including the patient, provider, regimen, and environment.[15].= It is also helpful to include some discussion of the HIV virus, HIV transmission, the HIV continuum of care or cascade, and biomedical and counseling therapies.
- *Person-centered, nonjudgmental counseling.* The MI approach focuses on acceptance and being nonjudgmental, as well as a neutral stance from the counselor when a participant is nonadherent with their antiretroviral medications. We also focus the discussion to emphasize the importance of *how* we say things over the content of *what* we say to our study participants.
- We found this approach to be supportive and helpful to MI clients, as many of them have never been asked about their experiences, their perspectives, and for their ideas on how best to adhere to their antiretroviral medications. In our model, we always assume that the participant is the expert of their own experience and that when the ideas and plans for adherence come from the participant, outcomes will be more sustainable. Our role as counselors is more to support and facilitate the

participant through the ambivalence they are likely experiencing and to explore the participants' values, what is important to them, and how confident they are in turning their adherence plan into a reality.

- *Supplemental materials to support the counselor in facilitating MI sessions.* We have developed and tested certain materials that are helpful in supporting counselors and clients, and often we review and practice with these materials in trainings. First, we teach counselors to use a standardized MI guide that includes all the steps of the research protocol and provides a sense of the flow of the session. Also included in this guide is specific language that the counselor can fall back on to use, if needed, especially during the sessions with the first few participants where the counselor is still gaining proficiency in session steps and flow. The guide can be helpful to make sure the counselors follow all of the steps, but the counselor is trained to view this tool as a guide rather than a script. This allows the counselor to follow their instincts and the MI spirit about where to go in a session even if it means skipping over a step or two. This guide also helps to have all of the counselors using the same resources for their sessions.

- Once the counselor has a good feel for the sessions, another resource we have found helpful is a data recording sheet (DRS). The DRS takes the more detailed guide and reduces it from a long document to a couple-page list. This document includes steps of the protocol and only key statements that the counselor can read, if needed. The DRS can allow the session to potentially have greater flow between the counselor and participant. Importantly, the DRS also serves as a place for the counselor to record steps they have completed, as well as responses made by the participant.

In an earlier chapter, the processes of MI were discussed. In the second MI process, that is, *focusing,* there are many ways to work with a participant related to medication adherence. One tool we have found beneficial to use is a *menu of options.* Such a menu of choices of topics to discuss typically will include numerous barriers and facilitators for the participant to pick from to explore in the session. Using the menu gives the participant autonomy to select a topic that is important to them and that will support them in considering the desired outcome of medication adherence. Using a menu of options also allows collaboration to occur and help equalize the counselor–participant power dynamic. An impromptu "brainstorming" session can also develop if the participant is having a challenging time coming up with ideas on their own. Lastly, looking at images or icons in a menu of options may be easier for a participant who has any literacy challenges.

"Mapping" can also be an important tool to consider to support alternative forms of learning. At the University of North Carolina–Chapel Hill, some research participants have preferred to *see* their thoughts put down in writing or to express themselves in more artistic or creative ways. This could include asking the participant to answer questions through diagraming rather than using words or crafting a combination of diagrams and words. When this approach is employed, asking the participant to interpret and discuss the meaning of their diagram is useful for many participants. This allows the participant to see more clearly how the past and present could influence future decisions. This technique was adapted from "node-link mapping" which has been used to augment counseling for drug abuse and other behaviors.[76]

Lastly, we have also incorporated other forms of media to support clients and counselors in MI interventions. For example, to help with explaining MI counseling to clients and obtaining buy-in, we have created DVDs and audio recordings featuring relatable characters role-playing different scenarios dealing with antiretroviral medication adherence and experiences of living with HIV. Clients and counselors can use examples from such media to facilitate their discussions, normalize behaviors, and conceptualize behavior change.

Ongoing Supervision and Coaching

In the third edition of *Motivational Interviewing: Helping People Change*, Bill Miller and Stephen Rollnick[74] discuss the importance of continued learning over time and, more specifically, individual feedback. Their recommendation is to focus less on attending workshops (after initial MI training) and more on receiving supervision/coaching. However, oftentimes this aspect of an MI intervention is overlooked due to competing demands and a sense of completion after the initial training.

At the University of North Carolina–Chapel Hill, our standard practice is to hire a clinical supervisor to provide regular support to MI counselors by allowing them to express their thoughts and feelings and raise questions in a safe environment. By having a neutral clinical supervisor who was otherwise not attached to the study, counselors could obtain guidance on working with their clients and strategies for increasing their MI proficiency and fidelity without fear of job-related consequences. Depending on the needs of the project and the counselors' caseloads, clinical supervision has been conducted with counselors as a group and/or individually, either in person or through Skype or conference call. Supervision sessions generally start with a check-in related to feelings and experiences that needed to be expressed and processed and then move into the presentation of cases, supplemented with audio or video recorded sessions if possible, and the review of relevant MI skills. It has been helpful to contract with clinical supervisors from outside our institution for the counselors to feel safe in disclosing their experiences, without the fear of being judged or evaluated by their respective employers.

Booster Training

A booster training has also been an important mechanism for enhancing the quality and fidelity of MI over time. After a predetermined or as-needed amount of time implementing the MI counseling intervention, our research project with HIV-positive inmates about to be released from prison had been going on for about a year, we conducted a booster training to allow counselors to develop a deeper understanding of the topics discussed in the original training. Conducting the booster after a year of implementation gave counselors the opportunity to share their experiences using MI skills with participants in real-world settings. In addition, time in the booster training provided the counselors a chance to role play and discuss specific situations they had encountered "in the field." The MI trainers also revisited effective strategies to work with individuals dealing with ART medication adherence and introduced new and advanced approaches to consider implementing.

Coding

Our last method of enhancing MI quality is using a behavioral coding system that determines how closely a clinician is using MI. Multiple coding systems have been developed and tested for the purpose of coding MI counselor and client behaviors and rating sessions for aspects of quality and fidelity.[63] In a recent meta-analysis of studies utilizing such coding systems, Magill[77] tested and partially validated a key causal model of MI efficacy in which therapist behaviors that are either consistent or inconsistent with MI correlate with client "change talk" (language in favor of behavior change), which mediated an overall effect on behavior change.[77] However, in a recent systematic review and meta-analysis of MI to reduce sexual risk behavior among PLWH, Naar-King[78] found that few studies utilized the "gold standard" of coding session recordings and concluded that future studies should consider using coding as a best fidelity practice.[78]

Two coding systems evaluating MI that we have used include the MITI code and the MISC; both are standardized systems intended for use as a treatment integrity measure for clinical trials and as a way to provide formal feedback to a clinician in a nonresearch setting. The MISC captures both clinician and client behaviors and their interactions, whereas the MITI measures only clinician behaviors. We used the MISC for earlier MI-based studies involving adherence[46] and safer sex practices[79] in which we found associations between MI quality and behavioral outcomes. Whether coding is used for research purposes, for supervision/coaching, or for skill development, starting coding early and continuing it in an ongoing manner is important. This allows a research project to determine the quality of delivery and can provide feedback if a clinician needs to increase proficiency. In the case of supervision/coaching and skill development, a baseline can be established, and a focus for additional training can be assessed. Training staff to perform MI coding can be time-consuming and resource-intensive, so it is advisable to budget accordingly.

FUTURE DIRECTIONS AND NEW MI TECHNOLOGIES

Using Technology to Support Delivery of MI for ART Adherence

Research on use of technology in supporting and enhancing health behaviors holds promise for the field of antiretroviral adherence. The use of technology to support or replace face-to-face evidence-based interventions may improve practitioners' ability to disseminate these interventions at lower cost to clients, particularly to those who face barriers to accessing in-person services (i.e., transportation or scheduling logistics) and/or frequently interact with technology in their daily lives. Medication adherence behaviors for chronic health conditions such as HIV may be particularly suited to technology-based interventions because taking medication is usually a daily behavior that spans a lifetime, a frequency and duration that is challenging to match with an in-person intervention. Furthermore, some researchers have used technology to deliver MI intervention components to promote health behaviors, suggesting that technology may hold promise as a mechanism of delivering MI to HIV-positive patients on ART.

Literature Relevant to the Use of Technology-Delivered MI Interventions for ART Adherence

Six recent systematic reviews[80–85] examined the use of technology-based interventions to promote ART adherence. Findings from these systematic reviews were consistently promising for technology-based interventions. Three reviews concluded that technology-based adherence interventions were acceptable and feasible among HIV-positive clients,[80,83,85] and all 6 found evidence of efficacy. Muessig et al.[84] identified 3 studies measuring the impact of mobile health interventions for ART adherence that showed increases in ART use intentions, self-reported adherence, and viral suppression, respectively. Devi et al.,[82] Amico et al.,[81] and Claborn et al.[80] found that the majority of technology-based intervention studies they identified demonstrated positive effects on ART adherence (33 of 47, 10 of 13, and 4 of 6, respectively). Finally, a meta-analysis by Daher[83] demonstrated that 4 SMS texting-based interventions significantly improved ART adherence (measured via MEMS caps) compared in RCT studies with controls (pooled odds ratio = 2.15, 95% confidence interval 1.18–3.91).

Out of these 6 reviews of ART adherence studies, only 2 individual studies[86,87] that used technology to deliver MI specifically were highlighted (in 4 of the 6 reviews),[80,81,83,85] and both of these individual studies targeted youth living with HIV. All 4 reviews highlighted the MESA study by Naar-King,[86] which used computer software to deliver 2 motivational intervention sessions to youth who had recently been prescribed ART. The computer software used an animated 2-dimensional character to deliver a realistic and brief conversational intervention, offering empathic reflections and emotional responses. Satisfaction ratings for the intervention were high, and effect sizes suggested that the intervention group showed a greater drop than controls in viral load from baseline to 6 months (Cohen's $d = 0.39$ at 3 months; $d = 0.19$ at 6 months) and had greater percentage undetectable by 6 months ($d = 0.28$). Effects sizes were medium to large for 7-day and weekend adherence. The Claborn et al.[80] review also identified the "+CLICK" intervention by Shegog et al.,[87] an innovative, Web-based, adherence intervention for HIV-positive youth as an adjunct to traditional clinic-based, self-management education. The application was developed for HIV-infected youth 13 to 24 years of age and based on concepts from social cognitive theory and MI and provided participants with tailored activities addressing attitudes, knowledge, skills, and self-efficacy related to ART adherence. Usability ratings indicated "+CLICK" was very easy to use (70%), trustworthy, and understandable (both >90%). Most (70%) indicated they would use "+CLICK" again. Short-term psychosocial outcomes indicate significant increase in medication adherence self-efficacy ($p < 0.05$), perceived importance of taking antiretroviral medicine close to the right time every day ($p < 0.05$), and knowledge about HIV and adherence ($p < 0.01$).

A small amount of additional evidence supporting technology-delivered MI is available in the non-HIV adherence literature. Kahwati et al.[88] reviewed 60 studies of medication adherence interventions for non-HIV medical conditions and identified several efficacious interventions that incorporated technology to promote adherence to self-administered medications for chronic diseases. Two studies specifically reported using technology in delivery of MI-based interventions: one used an automated telephone patient monitoring and counseling approach for adherence to antihypertensive medication and blood pressure control,[89] and the other study used a software-based counseling intervention provided over telephone for improving adherence to biological therapy among patients with multiple sclerosis.[90] Both interventions were automated or semiautomated, with no continuous professional support, and both led to improvements in medication adherence (as well as improvements in diastolic blood pressure in the antihypertensive study). One systematic review[91] of telephone-based IM studies for medication adherence identified 9 studies, 2 of which involved patients on medications to treat HIV.[54,58] The review found that while the heterogeneity of the studies hindered drawing definite conclusions, overall the authors thought their findings suggested that telephone-based MI may help improve medication adherence.

Another body of literature provides support for the use of technology in delivering MI-based interventions. A systematic review by Shingleton and Palfai[92] found 42 studies of MI interventions delivered with the help of technology to address a variety of health behaviors including substance use, risky sexual behaviors, and diet and physical activity. The review found that researchers have used a range of technologies such as chat rooms, automated computer responses, animated characters, emails, videos, and emoticons to deliver MI techniques including decision balances, readiness rulers, change plans, and open-ended questions. The technology used to deliver the MI-based intervention varied across studies in its degree of expert interaction (i.e., synchronous vs. asynchronous interaction or no expert communication) and level of media richness (e.g., text-only, audio files, video files). The results indicate that there is high acceptability of these interventions and, for studies that evaluated outcomes, generally consistent positive behavior change. However, the review authors note that studies were more likely to focus on delivering certain components of MI over others: strengthening commitment to change and developing discrepancy were more emphasized than aspects of MI spirit such as empathy and collaboration, possibly because the latter have fewer structured tools available for easy translation to technology. Also, the authors noted that studies rarely addressed adherence or quality of MI delivery using these technologies and suggest that researchers incorporate more traditional fidelity measures to help researchers understand whether or not the components of MI (both technical and relational) are being delivered adequately via technology

The great amount of recent literature on the use of technology to both promote adherence behaviors and administer MI interventions shows promise for the use of technology to deliver MI for ART adherence. Further research is needed to test this intervention method with HIV-infected adults and to incorporate indicators of MI fidelity.

Lessons Learned from SMS Technology for ART Adherence

As mentioned earlier, the imPACT intervention involved HIV-infected prisoners who were about to be released. The intervention spanned 8 to 12 weeks prerelease through 6 months postrelease. Our experience integrating SMS technology into this MI intervention for ART adherence was successful.

Upon release from prison, former prisoners received a cell phone. Text messages were sent to them for daily medication reminders. If desired by the participant, text messages could feature cloaked reminders (e.g., "Have a good day" vs. "Remember to take your HIV medication") to protect privacy. As well, text reminders were sent by study staff members to remind participants about clinic visits if they had not been reachable by phone, to conduct MI follow-up phone sessions, and to arrange face-to-face study visits by research assistants.

In imPACT, texts were well received, phones were provided feasibly, and sessions were both in-person and over the phone. However, there was still no effect on viral load.[93] In CARE-Plus, another study from the National Institute of Drug Abuse's Seek, Test, Treat and Retain research initiative with criminal justice system–involved populations, the researchers did a one-time interactive computerized MI session and SMS messaging via mobile phone with substance-using populations in jails. In the CARE-Plus study, a larger proportion of participants required replacement phones (58%) and over 90% did not turn in their smart phone as planned at the end of the study, indicating feasibility challenges. Despite these challenges, among the 110 study participants in the CARE+ trial, those in the CARE+ intervention arm had nearly twice the odds of viral suppression and slight increased odds of HIV care engagement compared with controls, although these finds were not statistically significant.[94] General challenges these studies identified in using technology with MI for HIV care adherence included reduced rapport with clients, difficulty in keeping in touch with people who may have inconsistent access to technology, and less control over ensuring a confidential, quiet, nondisrupted counseling setting.[95]

Peer-Delivered Interventions

Given the success of some peer-led interventions[96,97] in non-HIV settings[98–100] and for HIV prevention,[60,101] and an increasing attention being paid to identifying was to cost-effectively scale up effective adherence interventions, some researchers have begun to investigate the effectiveness of delivering MI-based interventions via peers,[102] including for addressing adherence to HIVcare.[55] Like MI, peer services are intended to be person-centered, nonjudgmental, and empathic.[102] Some MI-based programs for PLWH have combined peer education components with counselor-delivered MI but do not allow peers to deliver the MI,[54,103,104] but a few focus on peer delivery of MI. As Oh[102] indicates in his 2015 letter to *Psychiatric Services*, while core processes in the peer role are consistent with the principles of MI, for peers to adhere fully to MI processes, their interactions with clients would need to change, and little is known about their capacity to make such changes *or* the extent to which changes to accommodate MI processes might reduce other peer-counseling benefits. Oh points out that this is particularly true regarding peer counselor's self-disclosure behavior and suggests that more empirical evidence is needed to assess peer delivery of MI. Oh also indicates the importance of extensive training and supervision for peers to acquire and maintain MI skills. Oh's suggestions are consistent with studies to assess feasibility of peer-delivered counseling for ART adherence, including our own.[96,105] In one study by Wolfe et al.,[105] overall, peers had difficulty using open-ended questions and querying pros and cons, skills thought necessary to elicit change talk, and tended to give too much direct advice where reflections would have been appropriate. A challenge was training peers to change familiar ways of communicating. These findings were very consistent with those from our small pilot feasibility study in which the 6 peer counselors found the MI training to be acceptable and demonstrated the "spirit of MI," but their fidelity to MI quality was poor: peers had difficulty with reflecting and moving away from giving direct advice.[96] Until more studies are conducted to identify improved methods for training peers to conduct MI to address ART adherence and demonstrate efficacy are needed, we cannot say that there is evidence to support peer-delivered MI-based ART adherence interventions. As training methods are improved based on previous experience, however, peer-delivered MI may be found to be effective.

CONCLUSIONS

A strong rationale exists for the potential of using MI to counsel HIV-positive patients to adhere to their ART: the complex and variable nature of medication-taking and the individually tailored quality of MI suggest MI would be useful for this purpose. A narrative review of studies using MI to address ART adherence revealed that effective MI programs are delivered by MI-trained staff and place emphasis on measuring MI program fidelity. While most of the 13 studies we identified showed some positive effects of MI interventions on ART adherence, only 4 studies showed clear, consistent statistically significant results while most reported with null or mixed results, often due to insufficient power. Lessons learned from our own experiences delivering MI interventions indicate the importance of sufficient training from an experienced trainer who is a member of the MINT organization, ongoing coaching and supervision for the counselors, and a sufficient dose of MI for the clients based on providing MI for a sufficient duration and/or providing booster sessions and/or materials are important. Just as important is maintaining fidelity to the 4 processes of MI. Much recent attention has been paid to the use of technology to promote adherence behaviors and administer MI interventions. These studies suggest that there is promise for using technology to deliver MI for ART adherence but more research is needed before we will know if it works. This is an area of active research that those interested in MI should keep their eyes on. Similarly, in the last few years, several researchers have explored the possibility of peer delivery of MI, but several challenges have been identified that must be overcome and tested before robust evidence-based peer-delivered ART adherence interventions will be available. More research is needed to understand how best to use MI to address ART adherence. That said, it is clear that MI can offer an effective approach to adherence counseling for patients with HIV and that both MI quality—ensured via adequate training, supervision, and coding—as well as sufficient exposure to the intervention are critically important to its success.

REFERENCES

1. Feeney ER, Mallon PWG. HIV and HAART-associated dyslipidemia. *Open Cardiovasc Med J.* 2011;5:49–63. doi:10.2174/1874192401105010049
2. Enanoria WTA, Ng C, Saha SR, Colford JM. Treatment outcomes after highly active antiretroviral therapy: a meta-analysis of randomised controlled trials. *Lancet Infect Dis.* 2004;4(7):414–425. doi:10.1016/S1473-3099(04)01057-6
3. Bhaskaran K, Hamouda O, Sannes M, et al. Changes in the risk of death after HIV seroconversion compared with mortality in the general population. *JAMA.* 2008;300(1):51–59. doi:10.1001/jama.300.1.51
4. Bangsberg DR, Hecht FM, Charlebois ED, et al. Adherence to protease inhibitors, HIV-1 viral load, and development of drug resistance in an indigent population. *AIDS.* 2000;14(4):357–366.
5. Baeten JM, Donnell D, Ndase P, et al. Antiretroviral prophylaxis for HIV prevention in heterosexual men and women. *N Engl J Med.* 2012;367(5):399–410. doi:10.1056/NEJMoa1108524

6. Cohen MS, Chen YQ, McCauley M, et al. Prevention of HIV-1 infection with early antiretroviral therapy. *N Engl J Med.* 2011;365(6):493–505. doi:10.1056/NEJMoa1105243

7. Donnell D, Baeten JM, Kiarie J, et al. Heterosexual HIV-1 transmission after initiation of antiretroviral therapy: a prospective cohort analysis. *Lancet.* 2010;375(9731):2092–2098. doi:10.1016/S0140-6736(10)60705-2

8. Montaner JSG, Wood E, Kerr T, et al. Expanded highly active antiretroviral therapy coverage among HIV-positive drug users to improve individual and public health outcomes. *J Acquir Immune Defic Syndr.* 2010;55(Suppl 1):S5–S9. doi:10.1097/QAI.0b013e3181f9c1f0

9. Chandler RK, Kahana SY, Fletcher B, et al. Data collection and harmonization in HIV research: the seek, test, treat, and retain initiative at the national institute on drug abuse. *Am J Public Health.* 2015;105(12):2416–2422. doi:10.2105/AJPH.2015.302788

10. Lucas GM. Antiretroviral adherence, drug resistance, viral fitness and HIV disease progression: a tangled web is woven. *J Antimicrob Chemother.* 2005;55(4):413–416. doi:10.1093/jac/dki042

11. Chen LF, Hoy J, Lewin SR. Ten years of highly active antiretroviral therapy for HIV infection. *Med J Aust.* 2007;186(3):146–151.

12. Ying R, Barnabas RV, Williams BG. Modeling the implementation of universal coverage for HIV treatment as prevention and its impact on the HIV epidemic. *Curr HIV/AIDS Rep.* 2014;11(4):459–467. doi:10.1007/s11904-014-0232-x

13. Zablotska I. Ending the pandemic: reducing new HIV infections to zero. *J Int AIDS Soc.* 2013;16:18933. doi:10.7448/IAS.16.1.18933

14. Kato M, Long NH, Duong BD, et al. Enhancing the benefits of antiretroviral therapy in Vietnam: towards ending AIDS. *Curr HIV/AIDS Rep.* 2014;11(4):487–495. doi:10.1007/s11904-014-0235-7

15. Golin CE, Liu H, Hays RD, et al. A prospective study of predictors of adherence to combination antiretroviral medication. *J Gen Intern Med.* 2002;17(10):756–765.

16. Hudelson C, Cluver L. Factors associated with adherence to antiretroviral therapy among adolescents living with HIV/AIDS in low- and middle-income countries: a systematic review. *AIDS Care.* 2015;27(7):805–816. doi:10.1080/09540121.2015.1011073

17. Costa J de M, Torres TS, Coelho LE, Luz PM. Adherence to antiretroviral therapy for HIV/AIDS in Latin America and the Caribbean: Systematic review and meta-analysis. *J Int AIDS Soc.* 2018;21(1). doi:10.1002/jia2.25066

18. Ammassari A, Trotta MP, Murri R, et al. Correlates and predictors of adherence to highly active antiretroviral therapy: overview of published literature. *J Acquir Immune Defic Syndr.* 2002;31(Suppl 3):S123–S127.

19. Fogarty L, Roter D, Larson S, Burke J, Gillespie J, Levy R. Patient adherence to HIV medication regimens: a review of published and abstract reports. *Patient Educ Couns.* 2002;46(2):93–108.

20. Altice FL, Friedland GH. The era of adherence to HIV therapy. *Ann Intern Med.* 1998;129(6):503–505.

21. Wainberg MA, Friedland G. Public health implications of antiretroviral therapy and HIV drug resistance. *JAMA.* 1998;279(24):1977–1983.

22. Weidle PJ, Ganera CE, Irwin KL, et al. Adherence to antiretroviral medications in an inner-city population. *J Acquir Immune Defic Syndr.* 1999;22(5):498–502.

23. Murphy DA, Roberts KJ, Martin DJ, Marelich W, Hoffman D. Barriers to antiretroviral adherence among HIV-infected adults. *AIDS Patient Care STDS.* 2000;14(1):47–58. doi:10.1089/108729100318127

24. Chesney MA, Ickovics JR, Chambers DB, et al.; Patient Care Committee & Adherence Working Group of the Outcomes Committee of the Adult AIDS Clinical Trials Group (AACTG). Self-reported adherence to antiretroviral medications among participants in HIV clinical trials: the AACTG adherence instruments. *AIDS Care*. 2000;12(3):255–266. doi:10.1080/09540120050042891

25. Murri R, Ammassari A, Gallicano K, et al. Patient-reported nonadherence to HAART is related to protease inhibitor levels. *J Acquir Immune Defic Syndr*. 2000;24(2):123–128.

26. Catz SL, Kelly JA, Bogart LM, Benotsch EG, McAuliffe TL. Patterns, correlates, and barriers to medication adherence among persons prescribed new treatments for HIV disease. *Health Psychol*. 2000;19(2):124–133.

27. Holzemer WL, Corless IB, Nokes KM, et al. Predictors of self-reported adherence in persons living with HIV disease. *AIDS Patient Care STDS*. 1999;13(3):185–197. doi:10.1089/apc.1999.13.185

28. Kalichman SC, Ramachandran B, Catz S. Adherence to combination antiretroviral therapies in HIV patients of low health literacy. *J Gen Intern Med*. 1999;14(5):267–273.

29. Tuldrà A, Fumaz CR, Ferrer MJ, et al. Prospective randomized two-Arm controlled study to determine the efficacy of a specific intervention to improve long-term adherence to highly active antiretroviral therapy. *J Acquir Immune Defic Syndr*. 2000;25(3):221–228.

30. Gifford AL, Bormann JE, Shively MJ, Wright BC, Richman DD, Bozzette SA. Predictors of self-reported adherence and plasma HIV concentrations in patients on multidrug antiretroviral regimens. *J Acquir Immune Defic Syndr*. 2000;23(5):386–395.

31. Roberts KJ. Barriers to and facilitators of HIV-positive patients' adherence to antiretroviral treatment regimens. *AIDS Patient Care STDS*. 2000;14(3):155–168. doi:10.1089/108729100317948

32. Gordillo V, del Amo J, Soriano V, González-Lahoz J. Sociodemographic and psychological variables influencing adherence to antiretroviral therapy. *AIDS*. 1999;13(13):1763–1769.

33. Proctor VE, Tesfa A, Tompkins DC. Barriers to adherence to highly active antiretroviral therapy as expressed by people living with HIV/AIDS. *AIDS Patient Care STDS*. 1999;13(9):535–544. doi:10.1089/apc.1999.13.535

34. Meystre-Agustoni G, Dubois-Arber F, Cochand P, Telenti A. Antiretroviral therapies from the patient's perspective. *AIDS Care*. 2000;12(6):717–721. doi:10.1080/09540120020014255

35. Haynes RB, Taylor DW, Sackett DL. *Compliance in Health Care*. Baltimore, MD: Johns Hopkins University Press; 1979.

36. Miller WR, Rollnick S. *Motivational Interviewing: Preparing People for Change*. 2nd ed. New York, NY: Guilford Press; 2002.

37. Harding R, Dockrell MJ, Dockrell J, Corrigan N. Motivational interviewing for HIV risk reduction among gay men in commercial and public sex settings. *AIDS Care*. 2001;13(4):493–501. doi:10.1080/09540120120058021

38. Resnicow K, Jackson A, Wang T, et al. A motivational interviewing intervention to increase fruit and vegetable intake through Black churches: results of the Eat for Life trial. *Am J Public Health*. 2001;91(10):1686–1693.

39. Thevos AK. Motivational Interviewing enhances the adoption of water disinfection practices in Zambia. *Health Promot Int*. 2000;15(3):207–214. doi:10.1093/heapro/15.3.207

40. Kemp R, Kirov G, Everitt B, Hayward P, David A. Randomised controlled trial of compliance therapy. 18-month follow-up. *Br J Psychiatry.* 1998;172:413–419.

41. Burke BL, Arkowitz H, Menchola M. The efficacy of motivational interviewing: a meta-analysis of controlled clinical trials. *J Consult Clin Psychol.* 2003;71(5):843–861. doi:10.1037/0022-006X.71.5.843

42. Dunn C, Deroo L, Rivara FP. The use of brief interventions adapted from motivational interviewing across behavioral domains: a systematic review. *Addiction.* 2001;96(12):1725–1742. doi:10.1080/09652140120089481

43. Adamian MS, Golin CE, Shain LS, DeVellis B. Brief motivational interviewing to improve adherence to antiretroviral therapy: development and qualitative pilot assessment of an intervention. *AIDS Patient Care STDS.* 2004;18(4):229–238. doi:10.1089/108729104323038900

44. DiIorio C, McCarty F, Resnicow K, et al. Using motivational interviewing to promote adherence to antiretroviral medications: a randomized controlled study. *AIDS Care.* 2008;20(3):273–283. doi:10.1080/09540120701593489

45. Emmons KM, Rollnick S. Motivational interviewing in health care settings. Opportunities and limitations. *Am J Prev Med.* 2001;20(1):68–74.

46. Thrasher AD, Golin CE, Earp JAL, Tien H, Porter C, Howie L. Motivational interviewing to support antiretroviral therapy adherence: the role of quality counseling. *Patient Educ Couns.* 2006;62(1):64–71. doi:10.1016/j.pec.2005.06.003

47. Britt E, Hudson SM, Blampied NM. Motivational interviewing in health settings: a review. *Patient Educ Couns.* 2004;53(2):147–155. doi:10.1016/S0738-3991(03)00141-1

48. Centers for Disease Control and Prevention. HIV surveillance report, 2014. https://www.cdc.gov/hiv/pdf/library/reports/surveillance/cdc-hiv-surveillance-report-2014-vol-26.pdf. Published November 2015.

49. Pradier C, Bentz L, Spire B, et al. Efficacy of an educational and counseling intervention on adherence to highly active antiretroviral therapy: French prospective controlled study. *HIV Clin Trials.* 2003;4(2):121–131. doi:10.1310/hct.2003.4.2.007

50. Golin CE, Earp J, Tien H-C, Stewart P, Porter C, Howie L. A 2-arm, randomized, controlled trial of a motivational interviewing-based intervention to improve adherence to antiretroviral therapy (ART) among patients failing or initiating ART. *J Acquir Immune Defic Syndr.* 2006;42(1):42–51. doi:10.1097/01.qai.0000219771.97303.0a

51. Samet JH, Horton NJ, Meli S, et al. A randomized controlled trial to enhance antiretroviral therapy adherence in patients with a history of alcohol problems. *Antivir Ther.* 2005;10(1):83–93.

52. Parsons JT, Golub SA, Rosof E, Holder C. Motivational interviewing and cognitive-behavioral intervention to improve HIV medication adherence among hazardous drinkers: a randomized controlled trial. *J Acquir Immune Defic Syndr.* 2007;46(4):443–450.

53. Holstad MM, DiIorio C, Kelley ME, Resnicow K, Sharma S. Group motivational interviewing to promote adherence to antiretroviral medications and risk reduction behaviors in HIV infected women. *AIDS Behav.* 2011;15(5):885–896. doi:10.1007/s10461-010-9865-y

54. Konkle-Parker DJ, Erlen JA, Dubbert PM, May W. Pilot testing of an HIV medication adherence intervention in a public clinic in the Deep South. *J Am Acad Nurse Pract.* 2012;24(8):488–498. doi:10.1111/j.1745-7599.2012.00712.x

55. Naar-King S, Outlaw A, Green-Jones M, Wright K, Parsons JT. Motivational interviewing by peer outreach workers: a pilot randomized clinical trial to retain adolescents and young adults in HIV care. *AIDS Care.* 2009;21(7):868–873. doi:10.1080/09540120802612824

56. Jones DL, Sued O, Cecchini D, et al. Improving adherence to care among "hard to reach" HIV-infected patients in Argentina. *AIDS Behav.* 2016;20(5):987–997. doi:10.1007/s10461-015-1133-8

57. Goggin K, Gerkovich MM, Williams KB, et al. A randomized controlled trial examining the efficacy of motivational counseling with observed therapy for antiretroviral therapy adherence. *AIDS Behav.* 2013;17(6):1992–2001. doi:10.1007/s10461-013-0467-3

58. Cook PF, McCabe MM, Emiliozzi S, Pointer L. Telephone nurse counseling improves HIV medication adherence: an effectiveness study. *J Assoc Nurses AIDS Care.* 2009;20(4):316–325. doi:10.1016/j.jana.2009.02.008

59. Markham CM, Shegog R, Leonard AD, Bui TC, Paul ME. +CLICK: harnessing web-based training to reduce secondary transmission among HIV-positive youth. *AIDS Care.* 2009;21(5):622–631. doi:10.1080/09540120802385637

60. Outlaw AY, Naar-King S, Parsons JT, Green-Jones M, Janisse H, Secord E. Using motivational interviewing in HIV field outreach with young African American men who have sex with men: a randomized clinical trial. *Am J Public Health.* 2010;100(Suppl 1):S146–S151. doi:10.2105/AJPH.2009.166991

61. Madson MB, Loignon AC, Lane C. Training in motivational interviewing: a systematic review. *J Subst Abuse Treat.* 2009;36(1):101–109. doi:10.1016/j.jsat.2008.05.005

62. Miller WR, Moyers TB. Eight stages in learning motivational interviewing. *J Teaching Addictions.* 2006;5(1):3–17. doi:10.1300/J188v05n01_02

63. Madson MB, Campbell TC. Measures of fidelity in motivational enhancement: a systematic review. *J Subst Abuse Treat.* 2006;31(1):67–73. doi:10.1016/j.jsat.2006.03.010

64. Liu H, Golin CE, Miller LG, et al. A comparison study of multiple measures of adherence to HIV protease inhibitors. *Ann Intern Med.* 2001;134(10):968–977. doi:10.7326/0003-4819-134-10-200105150-00011

65. Hill S, Kavookjian J. Motivational interviewing as a behavioral intervention to increase HAART adherence in patients who are HIV-positive: a systematic review of the literature. *AIDS Care.* 2012;24(5):583–592. doi:10.1080/09540121.2011.630354

66. Golin CE, Earp JA, Grodensky CA, et al. Longitudinal effects of SafeTalk, a motivational interviewing-based program to improve safer sex practices among people living with HIV/AIDS. *AIDS Behav.* 2012;16(5):1182–1191. doi:10.1007/s10461-011-0025-9

67. Golin CE, Davis RA, Przybyla SM, et al. SafeTalk, a multicomponent, motivational interviewing-based, safer sex counseling program for people living with HIV/AIDS: a qualitative assessment of patients' views. *AIDS Patient Care STDS.* 2010;24(4):237–245. doi:10.1089/apc.2009.0252

68. Golin CE, Patel S, Tiller K, Quinlivan EB, Grodensky CA, Boland M. Start Talking About Risks: development of a Motivational Interviewing-based safer sex program for people living with HIV. *AIDS Behav.* 2007;11(5 Suppl):S72–S83. doi:10.1007/s10461-007-9256-1

69. Bandura A. Health promotion by social cognitive means. *Health Educ Behav.* 2004;31(2):143–164. doi:10.1177/1090198104263660

70. Fisher JD, Fisher WA. Changing AIDS-risk behavior. *Psychol Bull.* 1992;111(3):455–474. doi:10.1037/0033-2909.111.3.455

71. Fisher JD, Fisher WA, Bryan AD, Misovich SJ. Information-motivation-behavioral skills model-based HIV risk behavior change intervention for inner-city high school youth. *Health Psychol.* 2002;21(2):177–186. doi:10.1037/0278-6133.21.2.177

72. Fisher JD, Fisher WA, Misovich SJ, Kimble DL, Malloy TE. Changing AIDS risk behavior: effects of an intervention emphasizing AIDS risk reduction information, motivation,

and behavioral skills in a college student population. *Health Psychol*. 1996;15(2):114–123. doi:10.1037/0278-6133.15.2.114

73. Fisher JD, Fisher WA, Amico KR, Harman JJ. An information-motivation-behavioral skills model of adherence to antiretroviral therapy. *Health Psychol*. 2006;25(4):462–473. doi:10.1037/0278-6133.25.4.462

74. Miller WR, Rollnick S. *Motivational Interviewing: Helping People Change*. 3rd ed. New York, NY: Guilford Press; 2012.

75. Rollnick S, Mason P, Butler C. *Health Behavior Change: A Guide for Practitioners*. 2nd ed. Edinburgh, England: Churchill Livingstone; 2010.

76. Knight DK, Dansereau DF, Joe GW, Simpson DD. The role of node-link mapping in individual and group counseling. *Am J Drug Alcohol Abuse*. 1994;20(4):517–527.

77. Magill M, Gaume J, Apodaca TR, et al. The technical hypothesis of motivational interviewing: a meta-analysis of MI's key causal model. *J Consult Clin Psychol*. 2014;82(6):973–983. doi:10.1037/a0036833

78. Naar-King S, Parsons JT, Johnson AM. Motivational interviewing targeting risk reduction for people with HIV: a systematic review. *Curr HIV/AIDS Rep*. 2012;9(4):335–343. doi:10.1007/s11904-012-0132-x

79. Grodensky CA, Golin CE, Pack AP, et al. Adaptation and delivery of a motivational interviewing-based counseling program for persons acutely infected with HIV in Malawi: Implementation and lessons learned. *Patient Educ Couns*. 2018;101(6):1103–1109. doi:10.1016/j.pec.2018.02.004

80. Claborn KR, Fernandez A, Wray T, Ramsey S. Computer-based HIV adherence promotion interventions: a systematic review. *Transl Behav Med*. 2015;5(3):294–306. doi:10.1007/s13142-015-0317-0

81. Amico KR. Evidence for technology interventions to promote ART adherence in adult populations: a review of the literature 2012–2015. *Curr HIV/AIDS Rep*. 2015;12(4):441–450. doi:10.1007/s11904-015-0286-4

82. Devi BR, Syed-Abdul S, Kumar A, et al. mHealth: an updated systematic review with a focus on HIV/AIDS and tuberculosis long term management using mobile phones. *Comput Methods Programs Biomed*. 2015;122(2):257–265. doi:10.1016/j.cmpb.2015.08.003

83. Daher J, Vijh R, Linthwaite B, et al. Do digital innovations for HIV and sexually transmitted infections work? Results from a systematic review (1996–2017). *BMJ Open*. 2017;7(11):e017604. doi:10.1136/bmjopen-2017-017604

84. Muessig KE, LeGrand S, Horvath KJ, Bauermeister JA, Hightow-Weidman LB. Recent mobile health interventions to support medication adherence among HIV-positive MSM. *Curr Opin HIV AIDS*. 2017;12(5):432–441. doi:10.1097/COH.0000000000000401

85. Navarra A-MD, Gwadz MV, Whittemore R, et al. Health technology-enabled interventions for adherence support and retention in care among US HIV-infected adolescents and young adults: an integrative review. *AIDS Behav*. 2017;21(11):3154–3171. doi:10.1007/s10461-017-1867-6

86. Naar-King S, Outlaw AY, Sarr M, et al. Motivational Enhancement System for Adherence (MESA): pilot randomized trial of a brief computer-delivered prevention intervention for youth initiating antiretroviral treatment. *J Pediatr Psychol*. 2013;38(6):638–648. doi:10.1093/jpepsy/jss132

87. Shegog R, Markham CM, Leonard AD, Bui TC, Paul ME. "+CLICK": pilot of a web-based training program to enhance ART adherence among HIV-positive youth. *AIDS Care*. 2012;24(3):310–318. doi:10.1080/09540121.2011.608788

88. Kahwati L, Jacobs S, Kane H, Lewis M, Viswanathan M, Golin CE. Using qualitative comparative analysis in a systematic review of a complex intervention. *Syst Rev.* 2016;5:82. doi:10.1186/s13643-016-0256-y

89. Friedman RH, Kazis LE, Jette A, et al. A telecommunications system for monitoring and counseling patients with hypertension. Impact on medication adherence and blood pressure control. *Am J Hypertens.* 1996;9(4 Pt 1):285–292. doi:10.1016/0895-7061(95)00353-3

90. Berger BA, Liang H, Hudmon KS. Evaluation of software-based telephone counseling to enhance medication persistency among patients with multiple sclerosis. *J Am Pharm Assoc.* 2005;45(4):466–472.

91. Teeter BS, Kavookjian J. Telephone-based motivational interviewing for medication adherence: a systematic review. *Transl Behav Med.* 2014;4(4):372–381. doi:10.1007/s13142-014-0270-3

92. Shingleton RM, Palfai TP. Technology-delivered adaptations of motivational interviewing for health-related behaviors: A systematic review of the current research. *Patient Educ Couns.* 2016;99(1):17–35. doi:10.1016/j.pec.2015.08.005

93. Golin CE, Knight K, Carda-Auten J, et al. Individuals motivated to participate in adherence, care and treatment (imPACT): development of a multi-component intervention to help HIV-infected recently incarcerated individuals link and adhere to HIV care. *BMC Public Health.* 2016;16:935. doi:10.1186/s12889-016-3511-1

94. Kuo I, Liu T, Patrick R, et al. Use of a mHealth intervention to improve HIV treatment and engagement in HIV care among recently incarcerated persons in Washington, DC: a pilot study. *AIDS Behav.* 2019;23(4):1016–1031. doi:10.1007/s10461-018-02389-1

95. Christopoulos KA, Cunningham WE, Beckwith CG, et al. Lessons learned from the implementation of seek, test, treat, retain interventions using mobile phones and text messaging to improve engagement in HIV care for vulnerable populations in the united states. *AIDS Behav.* 2017;21(11):3182–3193. doi:10.1007/s10461-017-1804-8

96. Allicock M, Golin CE, Kaye L, Grodensky C, Blackman LT, Thibodeaux H. SafeTalk: training peers to deliver a motivational interviewing HIV prevention program. *Health Promot Pract.* 2017;18(3):410–417. doi:10.1177/1524839916663486

97. Gwadz MV, Collins LM, Cleland CM, et al. Using the multiphase optimization strategy (MOST) to optimize an HIV care continuum intervention for vulnerable populations: a study protocol. *BMC Public Health.* 2017;17(1):383. doi:10.1186/s12889-017-4279-7

98. Allicock M, Carr C, Johnson L-S, et al. Implementing a one-on-one peer support program for cancer survivors using a motivational interviewing approach: results and lessons learned. *J Cancer Educ.* 2014;29(1):91–98. doi:10.1007/s13187-013-0552-3

99. Allicock M, Haynes-Maslow L, Johnson L-S, et al. Peer Connect for African American breast cancer survivors and caregivers: a train-the-trainer approach for peer support. *Transl Behav Med.* 2017;7(3):495–505. doi:10.1007/s13142-017-0490-4

100. Paranjothy S, Copeland L, Merrett L, et al. A novel peer-support intervention using motivational interviewing for breastfeeding maintenance: a UK feasibility study. *Health Technol Assess.* 2017;21(77):1–138. doi:10.3310/hta21770

101. Hart TA, Stratton N, Coleman TA, et al. A pilot trial of a sexual health counseling intervention for HIV-positive gay and bisexual men who report anal sex without condoms. *PLoS One.* 2016;11(4):e0152762. doi:10.1371/journal.pone.0152762

102. Oh H. Peer-Administered motivational interviewing: conceptualizing a new practice. *PS.* 2015;66(5):558–558. doi:10.1176/appi.ps.201400583

103. Velasquez MM, von Sternberg K, Johnson DH, Green C, Carbonari JP, Parsons JT. Reducing sexual risk behaviors and alcohol use among HIV-positive men who have sex with men: a randomized clinical trial. *J Consult Clin Psychol.* 2009;77(4):657–667. doi:10.1037/a0015519

104. Gusdal AK, Obua C, Andualem T, et al. Peer counselors' role in supporting patients' adherence to ART in Ethiopia and Uganda. *AIDS Care.* 2011;23(6):657–662. doi:10.1080/09540121.2010.532531

105. Wolfe H, Haller DL, Benoit E, et al. Developing PeerLink to engage out-of-care HIV+ substance users: training peers to deliver a peer-led motivational intervention with fidelity. *AIDS Care.* 2013;25(7):888–894. doi:10.1080/09540121.2012.748169

8 Example Interventions Using Motivational Interviewing to Enhance Engagement in HIV Care

Laramie Smith, Riddhi Modi, and K. Rivet Amico

To reach the ambitious UNAIDS targets of 90% of people living with HIV reaching and sustaining viral suppression,[1] continuous engagement in antiretroviral therapy (ART) providing HIV care is critical. Evidence gathered to date suggests that a sizable minority of patients will experience gaps in treatment providing care,[2-4] even after linkage and access to ART. Less commonly, people may disengage entirely from ART providing HIV care.[5] Reasons for gapping identified to date include logistical issues (e.g., travel, move to a different region, changes in coverage or access to financial resources), social-motivational factors (e.g., negative experiences at point of care, high burden to attending care, feeling care is not of value or needed, high levels of surrounding HIV stigma), structural and personal costs of attending care, and low beliefs in benefits.[6-9] Models that attempt to organize experiences around engagement in HIV care include the situated information motivation behavioral skills model, Anderson's behavioral model, the socio-ecological model, and other applications of individual, social, and structural approaches.[8] Across models that organize potential drivers of sustained and continuous presentation in ART providing HIV care, motivation to engage in care is an essential component. As HIV-care clinics and sites engage in immediate ART start, experiment with novel strategies to facilitate easier schedules and ART access (e.g., move toward 6-month visit cycles, use of ART clubs where refills can be collected and then distributed in community), and implement differentiated patient care, the use of motivational interviewing (MI) to guide approaches is particularly timely to consider. We review two applications of MI in programs focused on optimizing engagement in care after linkage to care.

THE IENGAGE INTERVENTION

Developed to facilitate reaching viral suppression among those starting HIV-care within the first year of care, this intervention used an MI-based, counselor-delivered, face-to-face semistructured counseling approach supplemented by care appointment reminder calls.[10] As described in detail elsewhere,[10] the intervention integrated components of the Centers for Disease Control's Retention in Care

(RIC)[11,12] and Participating and Communicating (PACT) adherence intervention.[13] MI, used to guide the development and implementation of PACT, also was the basis for counselor–client interactions in iEngage. Aspects of MI utilized included spirit (i.e., partnership, acceptance, compassion and evocation), general processes (i.e., engaging, focusing, evoking, and planning), and training on general and specific communication strategies.[14]

As depicted in Figure 8.1, the iEngage intervention was delivered over the first year of HIV care through 4 face-to-face sessions with trained counselors, which coincided with regularly scheduled HIV-care visits. Between these visits, counselors placed calls to remind patients of upcoming HIV-care visits and followed up if a visit was missed. The main outcome for the study was 48-week viral suppression, and secondary outcomes included days to viral suppression and retention over time. Main findings for iEngage are expected for in the last half of 2019.

For each session, counselors focused on building strong relationships with patients through rapport building and fostering open communication. Each session followed a general flow, where exploration of current experiences and adjustment processes was followed by use of a screener assessment tool, adapted from RIC and enhanced to reflect challenges in early retention in care. Based on participant responses to whether or not certain concerns or barriers to returning for one's following HIV-care visit were reported, counselors created a plan for the remainder of the session that included activities (modules) that targeted those areas. The screener and modules used the situated information motivation behavioral skills (sIMB) model,[15] where knowledge, personal and social motivation, and skill sets were considered essential to optimize. Importantly, counselors worked with patients to understand how knowledge, beliefs, and strategies existed within one's current life context (i.e., structural, social, personal, and situational).

Across the 4 sessions, counselors provided HIV and ART education, with handouts and visual supports used as needed. When providing information, counselors were trained to use elicit–provide–elicit, such that patients were first asked what they understood about something and when more or different information was provided, counselors asked permission to share information, shared the information, and then asked patients about their interpretation of what was shared. In addition, the adjustment process that many people living with HIV go through after being diagnosis was included in education material using ideas from medical crisis counseling[16]—an approach the fosters autonomy and resilience. Each session also used a screener where items (questions) were asked of patients, and patients responded *yes* or *no* to a set of barriers to returning to care that were in the areas of organization, prioritization of

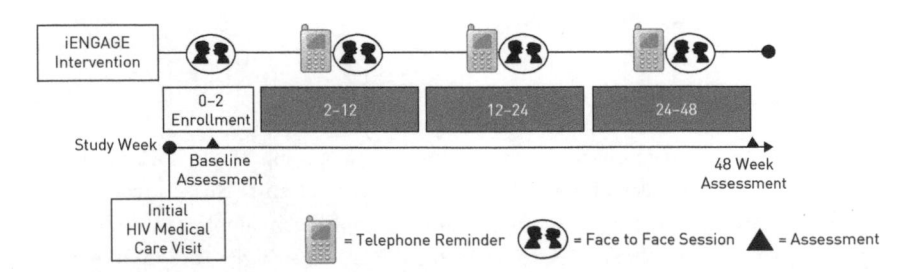

FIGURE 8.1. iEngage intervention overview.

self-care, communication with treatment team, treatment anxiety, negative affect, and problems that could benefit from referral to clinic resources (e.g., substance use, legal issues, finances, transportation). Concerns reported in any of these areas prompted counselors to use material from specific modules (Box 8.1) that all followed the same general process, although content varied. All modules concluded with goal planning, which was then summarized again at the end of the session.

Counselors were trained by behavioral scientists on the study team with support from trainers who practiced MI. As part of the training, the first skills highlighted were those common in MI, including use of reflections, summarizing, remaining affirming and nonjudgmental, emphasis on exploration, and promotion of patients identifying their own strategies and potential solutions. The intervention components in terms of screeners and modules were covered in trainings only after spirit and strategies to emulate MI spirit were discussed and practiced. In this manner, the foundation for the intervention was MI informed. However, it is important to note that some aspects of iEngage were separate from MI. Specifically, based on the evidence-based RIC and PACT interventions, iEngage sessions included a segment where counselors conducted an assessment of current unmet needs for returning to their next HIV care visit and, for those on ART, adherence, which was more directive in nature. Counselors had to move between a directive and guiding role as they moved through the intervention components in a given session. Although the intervention has not been evaluated from the perspective of the interventionists, this "ask" may have been challenging for counselors. Counselors were provided with a self-assessment tool that could be used to monitor spirit as well as fidelity to the overall iEngage approach. These were not used to collect data but rather as implementation tools. Fidelity in implementation was not included in the main trial.

Lessons learning in implementing a mixed intervention, where MI is used heavily but is not the core of the intervention, included challenges and advantages. In terms of challenges, it may have been challenging for counselors to be both directive and guiding in the same session and could have eroded patient autonomy. Using a screener and planned modules may have limited counselor flexibility in being able to engage in explorations or implement MI-based strategies as needed, which would arguably have been needed should change talk emerge during parts of the session that did not allow

---

Box 8.1

iEngage Screener and Intervention Modules

Screener Questions and Intervention Module Content Areas
Organization
Prioritization of Self Care
Communication with Treatment Team
Treatment Anxiety
Affect management/Problem Solving
Structural/resource challenges and referrals
Stigma
Disclosure

counselors to stop and explore it. However, counselors were trained to modify the session guide as needed, which may have addressed this limitation. It is also important to reiterate that fidelity and quality of sessions were not consistently documented. The intervention that is detailed in the intervention manual, procedures, and trainings, which depends heavily on MI strategies and principles. The intervention implemented may have drifted or been adapted in practice. The strengths of using MI in the intervention were readily apparent in facilitating training and providing counselors with a sound rationale and evidence base for using strategies that promote autonomy, partnership, and exploration and includes ways to work productively with resistance and foster change.

60 MINUTES FOR HEALTH INTERVENTION

In a single 60-minute session, the 60 Minutes for Health intervention draws on the past successes of brief theory-based single-session interventions to change HIV-related behaviors.[9-17] This format reflects the need for adaptable, low-resouce interventions that can be delivered at point of care when poorly retained patients engage with the HIV care system.[17] The intervention delivers a single, strong, targeted intervention dose to poorly retained people livng with HIV (PLWH). Intervention content is delivered using MI techniques[18] and was informed by a situated application of sIMB model.[19,20] The MI is used by the lay interventionist to target sIMB mechanisms of change that both facilitate retention in care and correct factors underlying decisions to delay or avoid HIV care.[20] These mechanisms are targeted via intervention activities that (i) identify and reduce misinformation guiding HIV care attendance; (ii) enhance motivation to maintain care via personal health goals; (iii) build skills for coping with negative feelings related to living with HIV; and (iv) increase self-efficacy for navigating structural barriers and to maintain HIV care amidst competing priorities. We discuss the formative work that guided the development of this intervention approach, how MI is leveraged to target mechanisms of change, and results from our randomized controlled pilot study of the intervention in the following text.

Formative Work

The development of the 60 Minutes for Health intervention drew extensively from our formative work with 20 tenuously engaged PLWH living in the Bronx, New York, the majority of whom had lifetime or recent experiences with structural barriers, substance use, and/or mental health. Results from our inductive and deductive analysis of participants' in-depth interviews highlighted critical contexts notably absent from the extant literature at the time, inlcuding (i) misinformation informing decisions to attend to, delay, or avoid HIV care—including the misperception that one is properly retained, (ii) motivation to engage in care for non-HIV related comorbidities, and (iii) motivation and behavioral skills to managing negative feelings towards living with HIV. Collectively, this work identified 7 theory-based mechanisms of change,[20] presented in Table 8.1, that the 60 Minutes for Health intervention seeks to target.

Table 8.1. Theory-Based Behavior Change Mechanisms Targeted in the 60 Minutes for Health Intervention

sIMB Intervention Targets to Improve Retention in HIV Care Behaviors	sIMB
1. Misinformation related to implicit rules (i.e., heuristics) guiding decisions to attend, delay or avoid HIV care (e.g., "I feel okay, so there is no reason to see my HIV doctor.")	I
2. Misinformation due to misperceptions that one "never miss appointments" or "doesn't go too long between doctor visits" despite documented gaps in care	I
3. Low motivation resulting from attitudes and beliefs that HIV care is a lower priority (i.e., HIV is more easily controlled) or being less concerned about HIV compared to other physical health conditions (e.g., diabetes, hypertension, cancer)	M
4. Low motivation resulting from personal beliefs and social normative attitudes that depression or active substance use negated their own or their provider's ability to address their HIV resulting in decisions to delay or avoid HIV care	M
5. Low motivation to stay engaged in care due to negative feelings about physical/emotional changes experienced in relation to living with HIV	M
6. Low behavioral skills (self-efficacy) for managing HIV care appointments when faced with structural barriers, competing priorities, non-HIV physical health comorbidities, and misinformation (as described in #1, #2, #3)	B
7. Low behavioral skills (self-efficacy) for managing social stigma and negative feelings about living with HIV related changes (#4, #5)	B

sIMB = situated information motivation behavioral skills.

Intervention Structure

60-Minutes for Health is a low-resource, clinic-based intervention to promote retention and HIV outcomes (i.e., viral load, CD4 count). Drawing on the past successes of brief theory-based, single-session interventions,[9–16] 60 Minutes for Health was designed to be delivered within the time and resource constraints of a busy HIV clinic setting. Using MI communication techniques,[18] the intervention is delivered by a lay health educator to poorly retained PLWH. This nonjudgmental, collaborative conversation positions the participant as the "expert" on the situations affecting their HIV care decisions. The health educator uses an illustrated workbook to guide the participant through the semistructured intervention activities during a 60-minute visit—the maximum billable time allowed for a health education session. The illustrated workbook was developed to be accessible to a range of literacy levels, while its "portability" minimizes disruptions to clinic activities. This flexibility allows the 60-minute intervention session to be implemented to patients presenting with a recent gap in HIV care in the clinic setting as soon as space and time are available. The low infrastructure and personnel resource burden of this intervention may enable future iterations of 60 Minutes for Health to potentially be delivered in community settings (e.g., library), removing the need for poorly retained PLWH to first come to the clinic.

MI-Delivered Intervention Content

The workbook contains 4 sections developed to identify and address critical sIMB deficits.[19,20] MI communicaiton techniques (i.e., OARS [open-ended questions, affirmations, reflective listening, summarizing] and Rolling with Resistance) are used to deliver intervention content and elicit change talk (i.e., DARN [desire, ability, reasons, and need for change], CAT [commitment, activation, and taking steps]) that reflect participants desire to change retention-related behaviors and plans for impimenting that change. Table 8.2 describes the time allocation, goals, activities, and theory-based mechanisms targeted in each section of the workbook. Examples from the pilot study depict how the lay health educator leveraged MI, across the 60 Mintues for Health workbook activities to tailor the intervention content to different participants and contexts affecting retention in HIV care.

Table 8.2. Review of 60 Minutes for Health Illustrated Workbook Activities Targeting and Theory-Based Mechanisms of Retention Behaviors

Workbook Sections, Time Allocations, and Activity Goals	*sIMB Model*	
1. Focusing on my physical health (10 min)		
Normalize and acknowledge retention in care challenges	I	B
Identify retention misinformation used to guide decisions to delay vs. attend HIV care visits	I	
Identify physical health priorities, and how they might be used to promote retention in HIV care	I	M
2. Focusing on my emotional health (20 min)		
Identify types of emotions, both positive and negative, participants feel about living with HIV	I	M
Help participants connect ways in which emotions affect how they engage in routine HIV care visits	M	B
Work to increase participants affect management self-efficacy[a]		B
3. Building on my HIV care history (15 min)		
Elicit contexts aiding or impeding retention in HIV care, including structural barriers such as transportation or health insurance	I	M
Develop a proactive plan for how to navigate similar situations to improve future retention behaviors	M	B
4. Achieving my personal health goals (15 min)		
Build on how participants see their physical/emotional health as relating to retention in care to identify a personal health goal	M	
Develop an action plan to help overcome barriers and reach that health goal in the next 6 months		B

[a]To strengthen these behavioral skills, participants are provided a printed instruction and an audio-CD containing brief affect management exercises to implement at home.

sIMBS =situated information motivation behavioral skills; I = targets retention-related (mis)information; M = targets personal/social motivations for attending HIV care; and B = identifies and strengthens retention-related behavioral skills.

Focusing on My Physical Health

This section targets ways indivudals may use information related to their HIV care, including misinformation, to guide their decisions to attend to, delay, or avoid HIV care. Specifically, the lay health educator starts the session using an image of the US treatment cascade to normalize retention as a challenging health behavior. This step is done to help reduce potential resistance from participants about discussing times they may have been poorly retained in HIV care. Next, images in the workbook facilitate the elicitaiton of information on HIV treatment knowledge and practices (e.g., how their provider refills ART prescriptions or monitors viral loads) to identify how (mis) information is used by the participant to guide their decisions to attend or delay visits ("If my doctor calls in a refill, its okay to skip this visit"). Finally, a 1-page immage depicting common HIV and non-HIV health comorbidities is then reviewed, eliciting discussion around current or future health priorities (e.g., diabetes, cancer). This is then used to elicit preparatory change talk around how routine visits with one's HIV care privider might help the participant to address these priorities ("I'm not worried about my HIV; it's my sugars that's gonna kill me").

Focusing on My Emotional Health

This section targets findings form our formative work that show how one feels about living with HIV can be a barrier to retention.[20] The lay health educator asks the participant to quickly sort 64 index cards into piles indicating how often living with HIV leads them to feel the emotion on each card (often, sometimes, never). Half of the cards are labeled with a postively valenced emotion (e.g., content, unbreakable, worthy). The other half are labeled with a negativly valenced emotion (e.g., exhasuted, reluctant, guilty). Using the emotions, the participant identified feeling often or sometimes, the lay health educator then guides the participant in a discussion to identify which feelings impact their decisions to attend, avoid, or delay care visits ("I feel exhausted when it's time to go to my doctor. It never ends. It's easier to curl up and take a nap"). They then discuss how brief affect-management skills have been used by similar others to cope with such emotions (e.g., breathing techniques, guided imagery, mindfulness meditations). The participant is then encouraged to select one of these brief affect-regulation skills to practice with the lay health educator. Each practice is approximately 5 mintues in length. The lay health educator then works to elicit implementation change talk to identify how and when the participant might work to build this skill set after this session. The particpant is provided with materials to practice and strengthen these skills at home (i.e., written practices in the workbook, a list of free apps that can be downloaded to a smart phone, and audio guided practices burned to a CD).

Building on My HIV Care History

This section is used to target 2 distinct theory-based determinants. First, it targets findings from our formative work that most poorly retained PLWH percieved themselves to be retained and actively invested in their HIV care, despite documentation in their medical records of having recently experienced substantial gaps in care (i.e., misinformation). And, second, it elicits sociostructural contexts that affects access to and engagment in medical care. In this seciton, the health educator uses an adapted timeline, follow-back method[18] to document the participants' HIV care history on an 18-month retrospective calendar, visibilly illustrating periods of time the participant went without a medical visit. To many participants, this discrepancy between their self-perception as someone who is engaged in their care and their medical records documented attended visits creates intrinsic motivation to improve on their current record. Using MI communicaiton techniques, the lay health educator further explores the participant's contexts, motivations, and behavioral skills related to times visits occurred (if any) and times they experienced a gap(s) in care ("I didn't want my doctor to know I relapsed and missed some meds"). This knowledge is used to develop a plan for navigating similar situations to improve retention behaviors ("I'll ask my doctor and social worker to meet me as a team at my next visits to support my recovery"). Upcoming visits are then written on a prospective 12-month calendar, identifying re-sources and personal strengths that could minimize past barriers if they were to occur again (i.e. skill building).

Achieving My Personal Health Goals

Finally, the information elicited through the previous workbook activities are summarized and used to explore how the participant views their physical and emo-tional health in light of retention-related motivations and behavioral skills ("I'm not worried about my HIV. I need to focus on my diabetes"). These insights are used to help the participant develop a personal health goal, eliciting from the par-ticipant, how this goal might be facilitated by maintaining more routine HIV care visits ("I'll write a list of what I eat each day when I take my ART and then talk with my doctor about how it affects my sugars"). The 60-minute session is then closed, using the workbook to develop an action plan to attain this goal in the next 6 months using the SMART goal principles (specific, measurable, achievable, rele-vant, and time-bound).

60 Minutes for Health Intervention Pilot

The 60 Minutes for Health intervention was then piloted in a sample of 16 poorly retained PLWH in the Bronx, New York, randomized 1:1 to receive either the 60 Minutes for Health intervention ($n = 8$) or the time-and-attention control session ($n = 8$) delivered via MI.[19] 60 Minutes for Health is acceptable and feasible to imple-ment.[19] Most participants were middle-aged ($M = 48.75$, $SD = 10.76$), female (62.5%), and identified as Hispanic/Latino (37.5%) or non-Hispanic black (62.5%). Immediately after their respective 60-minute session participants completed an acceptability and feasibility assessment.[21] Across both arms, participants favorably rated their respec-tive 60-minute session ($M = 4.75$, $SD = 0.45$; 1 = not favorable, 5 = very favorable). No significant ($p > 0.405$) or clinically meaningful differences were observed between participants' subjective experiences of their 60-minute session or perceived benefits of participation. All intervention activities were completed in the 60-minute timeframe.[21] Pilot results futher observed improved retention in HIV care (≥2 visits with an ART-monitoring provider >90 days apart in a 12-month interval).[21] Despite not being a

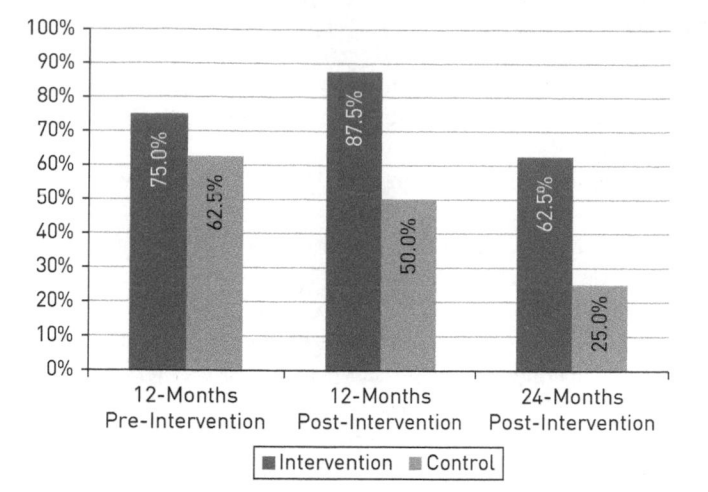

FIGURE. 8.2. Percentage retained in HIV care (Health Resources and Services Administration definition).

fully powered pilot study, more participants randomized to 60 Minutes for Health (vs. time-and-attention control) were retained in HIV care at 12 months (87.5% vs. 50.0%; p (2-tailed) = 0.282) and 24 months (62.5% vs. 25.0%; p (2-tailed) = 0.314) after receiving the intervention (see Figure 8.2). Findings suggest the intervention improved retention in care and was modestly protective against poorly retained PLWH dropping out of care over time.[21]

CONCLUSIONS

Each intervention described in this chapter is MI-informed, meaning that the spirit and specific strategies developed in MI were utilized in combination with other intervention strategies. Consistent between these interventions is the belief that patients ultimately have autonomy and self-determination, and interventionists are potentially effective guides in assisting patients to reach tailored goals by working with patients where they are, avoiding the righting reflex, and highlighting change talk when exploring ambivlance. The approaches prioritize compassion and exploration, while also actively guiding patients to reach their own conclusions. When working with PLWH in their navigation of what can be overwhelming systems of care, MI is particularly well-positioned to help clients to build skills, motivation, and commitment to developing and maintaining high engagement in HIV care.

CHAPTER NOTES

The iEngage intervention material are available upon request from the project PI (mmugavero@uabmc.edu). The 60 Minutes for Health intervention protocol and workbook materials are available upon request from the principal investigator (laramie@ucsd.edu). The chapter authors wish to thank all participants and study team members for iEngage and 60 Minutes for health.

REFERENCES

1. UNAIDS. 90-90-90: an ambitious treatment target to help end the AIDS epidemic. https://www.unaids.org/sites/default/files/media_asset/90-90-90_en.pdf. Published October 2014.

2. Mugavero MJ. Improving engagement in HIV care: what can we do? *Top HIV Med.* 2008;16(5):156–161.

3. Mugavero MJ, Amico KR, Horn T, Thompson MA. The state of engagement in HIV care in the United States: from cascade to continuum to control. *Clin Infect Dis.* 2013;57(8):1164–1171.

4. Mugavero MJ, Amico KR, Westfall AO, et al. Early retention in HIV care and viral load suppression: implications for a test and treat approach to HIV prevention. *J Acquir Immune Defic Syndr.* 2012;59(1):86–93.

5. Jose S, Delpech V, Howarth A, et al. A continuum of HIV care describing mortality and loss to follow-up: a longitudinal cohort study. *Lancet HIV.* 2018;5(6):e301–e308.

6. Giles M, MacPhail A, Bell C, et al. The barriers to linkage and retention in care for women living with HIV in an high income setting where they comprise a minority group. *AIDS Care.* 2019;31(6):730–736.

7. Hennink MM, Kaiser BN, Marconi VC. Pathways to retention in HIV care among US veterans. *AIDS Res Hum Retroviruses.* 2018;34(6):517–526.

8. Topp SM, Mwamba C, Sharma A, et al. Rethinking retention: mapping interactions between multiple factors that influence long-term engagement in HIV care. *PloS One.* 2018;13(3):e0193641.

9. Nabaggala MS, Parkes-Ratanshi R, Kasirye R, et al. Re-engagement in HIV care following a missed visit in rural Uganda. *BMC Res Notes.* 2018;11(1):762.

10. Modi R, Amico K, Knudson A, et al. Assessing effects of behavioral intervention on treatment outcomes among patients initiating HIV care: rationale and design of iENGAGE intervention trial. *Contemp Clin Trials.* 2018;69:48–54.

11. Gardner LI, Marks G, Shahani L, et al. Assessing efficacy of a retention-in-care intervention among HIV patients with depression, anxiety, heavy alcohol consumption and illicit drug use. *AIDS.* 2016;30(7):1111–1119.

12. Gardner LI, Metsch LR, Anderson-Mahoney P, et al. Efficacy of a brief case management intervention to link recently diagnosed HIV-infected persons to care. *AIDS.* 2005;19(4):423–431.

13. Golin CE, Earp J, Tien HC, Stewart P, Porter C, Howie L. A 2-arm, randomized, controlled trial of a motivational interviewing-based intervention to improve adherence to antiretroviral therapy (ART) among patients failing or initiating ART. *J Acquir Immune Defic Syndr.* 2006;42(1):42–51.

14. Miller WR, Rollnick S. *Motivational Interviewing: Helping People Change.* New York, NY: Guilford Press; 2012.

15. Amico K. A situated-information motivation behavioral skills model of care initiation and maintenance (sIMB-CIM): an IMB model based approach to understanding and intervening in engagement in care for chronic medical conditions. *J Health Psychol.* 2011;16(7):1071–1081.

16. Pollin I, Kanaan SB. *Medical Crisis Counseling: Short-Term Therapy for Long-Term Illness.* New York: W. W. Norton; 1995.

17. Smith LR, Amico KR, Shuper PA, et al. Information, motivation, and behavioral skills for early pre-ART engagement in HIV care among patients entering clinical care in KwaZulu-Natal, South Africa. *AIDS Care.* 2013;25(12):1485–1490.

18. Sobell LC, Sobell MB. Timeline follow-back. In: Litten RZ, Allen JP, eds. *Measuring Alcohol Consumption*. New York: Springer; 1992: 41–72.

19. Smith LR, Amico KR, Fisher JD, Cunningham CO. 60 Minutes for health: examining the feasibility and acceptability of a low-resource behavioral intervention designed to promote retention in HIV care. *AIDS Care*. 2018;30(2):255–265.

20. Smith LR, Fisher JD, Cunningham CO, Amico KR. Understanding the behavioral determinants of retention in HIV care: a qualitative evaluation of a situated information, motivation, behavioral skills model of care initation and maintenance. *AIDS Patient Care and STDs*. 2012;26(6):344–355.

SECTION III
APPLICATIONS OF MOTIVATIONAL INTERVIEWING IN ADDRESSING COMORBID CONDITIONS

9 Lifestyle Changes and Motivational Interviewing

David A. Martinez and
Sofie L. Champassak

BACKGROUND

To adequately manage and prevent HIV disease, it is important to address lifestyle behaviors such as substance use and risky sexual behaviors.[1-4] Although not one single definition for risky sexual behavior is agreed on by all health entities, usually risky sexual behaviors are considered as sexual behaviors that increase the chance of a negative outcomes, such as condomless sex, multiple partners, sex under the influence of drug and alcohol, IV drug use, paying for sex, and untreated sexually transmitted illness, among others. It is also important to open conversations around factors, decisions, habits, and substance use that lead to other chronic health issues (i.e., smoking) among people living with HIV (PLWH). Motivational interviewing (MI) has been shown to be an effective and brief approach to reduce sexual risk behaviors (condomless sex), substance use, and smoking.[3,5-7] This chapter serves as a brief, practical, evidence-based MI guide for practitioners to address particular behaviors and issues that place PLWH at increased risk for poor health outcomes.

As we have discussed earlier in the book, MI is a "collaborative, goal-oriented style of communication with particular attention to language of change, designed to strengthen personal motivation for and commitment to a specific goal by eliciting and exploring the person's own reasons for change within an atmosphere of acceptance and compassion ."[8p29] MI is defined by its spirit of collaboration, compassion, acceptance, and evocation and employs open-ended skills such as open-ended questions, affirmations, reflections, and summaries (OARS) to accomplish its goals.

SUBSTANCE USE AND TOBACCO USE

Substance use behaviors and disorders are common among PLWH[1,9] and can negatively impact their health and quality of life. For example, substance use may accelerate disease progression[10-12] and increase complications of HIV disease, including co-occurring illnesses such as tuberculosis, hepatitis C, and depression.[13,14] Using substances may also negatively impact medication adherence.[15-18]

Routine alcohol, tobacco, and illicit substance use screenings are encouraged in the primary care setting[19,20] and should be included with routine HIV care as PLWH have higher rates of using tobacco, alcohol, and illicit substances.[5] However, many practitioners fail to comply with this recommendation.[21,22] Further, screening may identify issues but do not necessarily assist practitioners in having productive conversations about them with patients. Barriers that prevent primary care practitioners from having discussions about substance use with their patients include factors related to both the practitioner and the patient.[23] Practitioners have expressed system-level concerns such as lack of time, space, resources, and individual-level concerns such as limited substance use knowledge and training. Patients have reported concerns about confidentiality and consequences related to disclosing substance use.[24]

MI has been shown to reduce substance use and improve medication adherence for PLWH.[5] When focused on benefits of behavior change or planning for change, rather than current behavior pattern, patients are more likely to voice change talk, a key strategy of MI, related to alcohol use and other problematic behaviors.[25] In the following discussion we provide examples of MI-consistent approaches and statements to discuss alcohol and substance use behaviors with patients.[8]

As illustrated in the following clinical case, it is important to facilitate a discussion about substance use and enhance motivation for change using open-ended questions, affirmations, reflections, and summaries (OARS), particularly reflections, to help patients elaborate about their use, identify how their use may be affecting their health, and maintain the spirit of collaboration.

The patient is a 32-year-old woman who was diagnosed with HIV 2 years ago. She stopped using methamphetamines 5 years ago. During her initial appointment, she stated that she is a "social drinker and smoker." The patient states that she drinks between 5 to 9 cocktails about 1 to 2 days a week and occasionally does not remember some of the events from the night before. She does not believe that her alcohol use is problematic, and she feels ambivalent about decreasing her alcohol use. She attends all her medical appointments and has expressed concerned about her high viral load.

Practitioner: Welcome. You're always on time and you have made all effort to attend all your appointments with me. (Affirmation)

Patient: Yeah, I guess so, and my viral load hasn't improved.

Practitioner: You are worried about your viral load not improving despite being in treatment. What do you think contributes to the high viral load? (Reflection followed by an open-ended question)

Patient: Well, I'm trying to take care of myself and take my medications as recommended.

Practitioner: You are adhering to your medications since your health is important to you. What's been like taking the medications? (Reflection followed by an open-ended question)

Patient: Well, I take them when I'm supposed to, but I guess sometimes I forget maybe a couple times a week.

Practitioner: You are trying to take them consistently and at the same time you miss 2 doses a week. (Reflection)

Patient: Sometimes I'm hanging out with my friends drinking, and I just lose track of time or don't have 'em on me.

Practitioner: Your drinking makes it harder for you to stick to them as recommended. (Reflection)

Patient: Yeah, sometimes, it's not all the time.

Practitioner: You don't see it as a major issue for you. (Reflection)

Patient: I don't think so. I mean I drink like once a week.

Practitioner: You don't think it's a problem, and just sometimes your drinking causes you to forget to take your medications. How else does having few drinks affect you? (Reflection followed by an open-ended question)

Patient: I start feeling more relaxed, confident, like nothing's wrong with me.

Practitioner: Drinking makes you feel less anxious and invincible. (Reflection)

Patient: Yeah, but the next day I feel horrible, and then I forget to take my meds, and here I am with the same viral load, and I am worried about my health.

Practitioner: You want to have better control over your illness. (Reflection)

Patient: Yeah, of course.

Practitioner: What do you think you could do differently? (Evocative question)

Patient: I probably need to keep better track of taking my meds.

Practitioner: You need to make sure to not miss any doses of your meds. (Reflection)

Patient: Well, I usually forget because I've been drinking.

Practitioner: So clearly your drinking interferes with your ability to take your medications. (Reflection)

Patient: Yes, but I like drinking, I also see how it's affecting my health. I just don't know how or where to start.

Practitioner: You are conflicted about what to do at this time. How do you feel about discussing some options regarding your drinking and strategies to help you stay adherent to your meds and then you can decide what works best for you? (Reflection followed by asking permission about a menu of options)

Patient: Sure, I guess that's a good place to start.

USING OARS TO DISCUSS A PATIENT'S SUBSTANCE USE

Open-ended questions that invite the patient to provide additional information about their use and cannot be answered with a one-word answer (e.g., "yes" or "no"). Examples of open-ended questions include the following.

"How do you feel about the amount you're drinking?"
"How does your smoking impact your health?"
"What do you think would be most helpful for you right now?"

Affirmations are statements that help convey understanding and appreciation. These statements can build or sustain rapport with a patient. Examples of affirmations include the following.

"It can be difficult to talk about this. I appreciate your willingness to have this discussion."
"You want things to be different and are really trying to make a change."
"You value you're being health."

Reflections are statements that demonstrate understanding or can be used to elicit additional information for clarification. These statements can include the patient's words, meanings, and or feelings expressed during your discussion. Examples of reflections include the following.

"You enjoy using and it's not causing you any problems."
"You're tired of hearing the same thing from your doctors about your smoking."
"You feel really overwhelmed."

Summaries are a collection of concise statements that are pulled together from the discussion and are used throughout the discussion. The statements are selectively chosen to highlight parts of your discussion to demonstrate that you have been listening, can assist the patient to elaborate further, or can assist the patient to transition to the next topic.

An example of a summary is as follows.

"You think drinking is fun and helps you to relieve stress. You mentioned that sometimes you make riskier choices when you're drunk like having unprotected sex and also forgetting to take your medications. You value your health and want to make changes, and you're unsure of where to start."

SEXUAL BEHAVIORS THAT MAY INCREASE RISKS FOR TRANSMISSION OR INFECTION

Prior to the advent of treatment for prevention, efforts to provide education and support to PLWH to reduce condomless sex events or other sexual behaviors that could transmit HIV based in MI were evaluated and had some success. MI has demonstrated effectiveness in some of these evaluations. One study reported that an increase in the amount of MI minutes received by patients was associated with a decrease in condomless sex among PLWH, including youth and older adults[3,4,6,7,26] A key to behavior change is to increase self-efficacy. Increases in self-efficacy to practice safer sex has been associated with a higher number of MI sessions such that MI may increase an individual's own belief that they are able to engage in safer sex practices.[2] Furthermore, the use of reflective listening is a central tool to MI. Higher frequency of reflections has predicted fewer condomless sex events among PLWH.[27] MI's effectiveness for increasing condom use or decreasing unprotected sex among MSM is unclear.[28] However, having a conversation with all patients about sexual health is better than not addressing it at all.

As illustrated in the following case, to increase motivation for change, it is important to help the patient explore his ambivalence about change by developing discrepancy between his sexual behavior and his goals/values.

The patient is a 45-year-old man who was diagnosed HIV-positive 15 years ago. He is prescribed antiretroviral therapy (ART), struggles with adherence, and has a history of unsuppressed viral load. He has been abstinent from heavy alcohol and methamphetamine use for the past 5 years. He is currently in a serious relationship and engages in sexual intercourse with casual partners occasionally. He reports he does not use condoms with partners who are HIV-positive. His primary care physician referred him to the therapist in the clinic to have a conversation about his understanding of his behaviors. In the first brief encounter, the therapist reviewed with the patient his thoughts about his unprotected sex practices, assessed the patient's motivation for change, and explored his ambivalence about his current behaviors.

Practitioner: What is your understanding of the reasons your doctor referred you to see me? (Open-ended question)

Patient: He would like me to discuss some of my sexual behaviors.

Practitioner: Is it okay with you to have a conversation about things going on with you? I think more about things going on sexually, if that's okay? (Asking permission)

Patient: Sure.

Practitioner: You mentioned earlier that you enjoy sex without condoms right now. (Reflection)

Patient: Well, only sometimes, and I only do it with people who have HIV.

Practitioner: You don't have sex without condom all the time. (Reflection)

Patient: Yeah, it's not a big deal, right?

Practitioner: You are wondering whether you should be concerned about having sex without using a condom with people who have HIV. (Reflection)

Patient: Well, if they're infected, then I can't infect them either. And having sex with no condom feels so much better. But, maybe, I should be more careful. I use condoms with people that don't have HIV. Plus, I have an undetectable viral load.

Practitioner: So you're being safe just with people that you believe don't have HIV. (Reflection)

Patient: Yeah, if I use condoms with people who are not sick, I won't spread it. Isn't that true?

Practitioner: I can share my thoughts if it is okay with you. (Asking permission)

Patient: Sure. I need to know whether I am taking any risk because I do not want to mess up my viral load.

Practitioner: Sex without condom among individuals with HIV comes with a certain low risk, which is getting infected with a new distinct HIV viral strain and acquiring other STDs. What do you think? (Sharing information followed by an open-ended question)

Patient: I'm tired of having to worry about using condoms all the time. But I know that's what I am supposed to do, I mean to play it safely, but I just want a break sometimes.

Practitioner: Sometimes you don't want to stick to safer sex practices, and at the same time you are very much aware of consequences of not using condoms all the time. (Reflection)

Patient: Of course, I know the risks very well. I know that I can contract other STDs or give one to my sexual partners.

Practitioner: You also care about your own health. (Reflection)

Patient: Oh, yes, of course.

Practitioner: How would you like to proceed with any changes of your behaviors at this time? (Evocative question)

The previous case illustrates the exploration of the patient's ambivalence about changing his risky sexual behavior. Rather than prematurely focusing on the patient's belief that engaging in unprotected sex with other people with HIV was low risk, the practitioner sought to understand the reasons why it would be important for him to change.

MI is not a comprehensive treatment approach, but it is a tool to help patients resolve ambivalence in the direction of change.[8] For that reason, MI can be used in combination with other practical treatment approaches (e.g., cognitive behavioral therapy or other behavioral interventions) when helping patients make plans to reduce their sexual risk taking and substance use. Lastly, when patients receive MI, they are more likely to change multiple behaviors simultaneously, like improve ART adherence and decrease sexual risk.[29]

REFERENCES

1. Bing EG, Burnam MA, Longshore D, et al. Psychiatric disorders and drug use among human immunodeficiency virus–infected adults in the United States. *Arch Gen Psychiatry.* 2001;58(8):721–728.

2. Chariyeva Z, Golin CE, Earp JA, Suchindran C. Does motivational interviewing counseling time influence HIV-positive persons' self-efficacy to practice safer sex?. *Patient Educ Couns.* 2011;87(1):101–107.

3. Chen X, Murphy DA, Naar-King S, Parsons JT. Adolescent Medicine Trials Network for HIV/AIDS Interventions: a clinic-based motivational intervention improves condom use among subgroups of youth living with HIV. *J Adolesc Health.* 2011;49(2):193–198.

4. Fisher JD, Cornman DH, Shuper PA, et al. HIV prevention counseling intervention delivered during routine clinical care reduces HIV risk behavior in HIV-infected South Africans receiving antiretroviral therapy: the Izindlela Zokuphila/Options for Health randomized trial. *J Acquir Immune Defic Syndr.* 2014;67(5):499–507.

5. Durvasula R, Miller TR. Substance abuse treatment in persons with HIV/ AIDS: challenges in managing triple diagnosis. *Behav Med.* 2014;40(2):43–52.

6. Chariyeva Z, Golin CE, Earp JA, Maman S, Suchindran C, Zimmer C. The role of self-efficacy and motivation to explain the effect of motivational interviewing time on changes in risky sexual behavior among people living with HIV: a mediation analysis. *AIDS Behav.* 2013;17(2):813–823.

7. Lovejoy TI, Heckman TG, Suhr JA, et al. Telephone-administered motivational interviewing reduces risky sexual behavior in HIV-positive late middle-age middle aged and older adults: a pilot randomized controlled trial. *AIDS Behav.* 2011;15(8):1623–1634.

8. Miller WR, Rollnick S. *Motivational Interviewing: Helping People Change.* 3rd ed. New York, NY: Guilford Press; 2013.

9. Rabkin JG, McElhiney MC, Ferrando SJ. Mood and substance use disorders in older adults with HIV/AIDS: methodological issues and preliminary evidence. *AIDS.* 2004;18:43–48.

10. Carrico AW. Substance use and HIV disease progression in the HAART era: implications for the primary prevention of HIV. *Life Sci.* 2011;88(21-22):940–947.

11. Kipp AM, Desruisseau AJ, Qian HZ. Non-injection drug use and HIV disease progression in the era of combination antiretroviral therapy. *J Subst Abuse Treat.* 2011;40(4):386–396.

12. National Institute on Alcohol Abuse and Alcoholism. Effects on the immune system. https://pubs.niaaa.nih.gov/publications/10report/chap04b.pdf. Published 2010.

13. Centers for Disease Control and Prevention. Integrated prevention services for HIV infection, viral hepatitis, sexually transmitted diseases, and tuberculosis for persons who use drugs illicitly: summary guidance from CDC and the U.S. Department of Health and Human Services. *MMWR.* 2012 Nov 9;61(RR05);1–40. https://www.cdc.gov/mmwr/preview/mmwrhtml/rr6105a1.htm.

14. Levintow SN, Pence BW, Ha TV, et al. Prevalence and predictors of depressive symptoms among HIV-positive men who inject drugs in Vietnam. *PLoS One.* 2018;13(1):e0191548. doi:10.1371/journal.pone.0191548

15. Azar MM, Springer SA, Meyer JP, Altice FL. A systematic review of the impact of alcohol use disorders on HIV treatment outcomes, adherence to antiretroviral therapy and health care utilization. *Drug Alcohol Depend.* 2010;112(3):178–193.

16. Hinkin CH, Barclay TR, Castellon SA, et al. Drug use and medication adherence among HIV-1infected individuals. *AIDS Behav.* 2007;11(2):185–194.

17. Kalichman SC, Grebler T, Amaral CM, et al. Viral suppression and antiretroviral medication adherence among alcohol using HIV-positive adults. *Int J Behav Med.* 2014;21(5):811–820.

18. Parsons JT, Rosof E, Mustanski B. The temporal relationship between alcohol consumption and HIV-medication adherence: a multilevel model of direct and moderating effects. *Health Psychol.* 2008;27(5):628–637.

19. Substance Abuse and Mental Health Services Administration. The case for behavioral health screening in HIV care settings. HHS Publication No. SMA-16-4999. Rockville, MD: Substance Abuse and Mental Health Services Administration. https://store.samhsa.gov/system/files/sma16-4999.pdf.

20. U.S. Preventive Services Task Force. Final recommendation statement: alcohol misuse: screening and behavioral counseling interventions in primary care. https://www.uspreventiveservicestaskforce.org/Page/Document/UpdateSummaryFinal/alcohol-misuse-screening-and-behavioral-counseling-interventions-in-primary-care. Published May 2013.

21. Dawson-Rose C, Draughon JE, Zepf R, et al. Prevalence of substance use in an HIV primary care safety net clinic: a call for screening. *J Assoc Nurses AIDS Care.* 2015;28(2):238–249.

22. Surah S, Kieran J, O'Dea S, et al. Use of the Alcohol Use Disorders Identification Test (AUDIT) to determine the prevalence of alcohol misuse among HIV-infected individuals. *Int J STD AIDS.* 2013;24(7):517–521.

23. McNeely J, Kumar PC, Rieckmann T, et al. Barriers and facilitators affecting the implementation of substance use screening in primary care clinics: a qualitative study of patients, providers, and staff. *Addict Sci Clin Pract.* 2018;13(1):8. doi:10.1186/s13722-018-0110-8

24. Ray MK, Beach MC, Nicolaidis C, Choi D, Saha S, Korthuis PT. Patient and provider comfort discussing substance use. *Fam Med.* 2013;45(2):109–117.

25. Kahler CW, Caswell AJ, Laws MB, et al. Using topic coding to understand the nature of change language in a motivational intervention to reduce alcohol and sex risk behaviors in emergency department patients. *Patient Educ Couns.* 2016;99(10):1595–1602.

26. Goggin K, Gerkovich MM, Williams KB, et al. A randomized controlled trial examining the efficacy of motivational counseling with observed therapy for antiretroviral therapy adherence. *AIDS Behav.* 2013;17(6):1992–2001.

27. Grodensky C, Golin C, Parikh MA, et al. Does the quality of SafeTalk motivational interviewing counseling predict sexual behavior outcomes among people living with HIV?. *Patient Educ Couns.* 2016;100(1):147–153.

28. Berg RC, Tikkanen R, Ross NW. Motivational interviewing for HIV-related behaviors among men who have sex with men. Report no. 2011-17. Oslo, Norway: Norwegian Knowledge Centre for Health Services; 2011.

29. Holstad MM, DiIorio C, Kelley ME, Resnicow K, Sharma S. Group motivational interviewing to promote adherence to antiretroviral medications and risk reduction behaviors in HIV infected women. *AIDS Behav.* 2011;15(5):885–896.

10 Comorbid Medical Problems and Motivational Interviewing

Sharon Connor and Hanna K. Welch

BACKGROUND

Deaths from HIV infection have greatly declined in the United States since the 1990s. Worldwide, the lifespan for people with HIV is longer due to the scale-up of antiretroviral therapy (ART) in developing countries.[1] Due to increasingly effective treatments for HIV, people living with HIV (PLWH) are living healthier and more productive lives. Longer lifespans require an emphasis on maintaining quality and length of life in patients.

It is important to consider the health and wellness goals that apply for all people. In the United States, the health agenda for the nation, Healthy People 2020, includes the overarching goals that describe the ability of all people to attain high-quality, longer lives free of preventable disease, disability, injury, and premature death.[2] Included in these goals are health equity, the elimination of disparities, and the opportunity to improve the health of all.[2] Important considerations must be made for PLWH as they age and face multiple chronic diseases. Optimal care requires a multifaceted team.

HIV AND COMMON COMORBID MEDICAL PROBLEMS

Chronic disease is common in all populations as they age. In fact, diabetes, cancer, cardiovascular disease, and other chronic conditions account for most deaths in high-income, middle-income, and many lower middle-income countries.[3] Besides causing early death, chronic disease impacts the quality of life of individuals.[4] Although people are living longer, they are not necessarily healthier. This long-term burden of illness and diminished well-being affects patients, families, health systems, and economies.

Co-morbid conditions increase the complexity of care when managing the health of PLWHA.[5] There are estimates that by the year 2030, a majority of PLWH will be over the age of 50, resulting in a larger population at a higher risk for multiple co-morbidities.[6] The management of chronic disease must be optimized if PLWH are to live healthy lives. The care of PLWH must be integrated to include the management of both communicable and non-communicable diseases.[3] Moreover, the World Health Organization says, "Ageing well must be a global priority."[7]

This is an urgent matter particularly in terms of higher risks for ischemic heart disease and congestive heart failure,[8,9] hypertension,[6] and diabetes[10] among PLWH. Additionally, 20% to 30% of PLWH in the United States are co-infected with hepatitis C virus.[11] Moreover, the medications used to treat HIV may contribute to chronic disease such as type 2 diabetes and hyperlipidemia.[12,13] The World Health Organization has noted the inability of current health care systems to address the burden of chronic disease.[7] Leaders note the challenge of treating patients optimally when faced with co-morbid medical problems.[14,15]

MOTIVATIONAL INTERVIEWING AND ITS INFLUENCE ON THE ABILITY TO MANAGE CHRONIC DISEASE

Patient-centered care is a key component of chronic disease management. In patient-centered care, patients' values and beliefs are incorporated into the care plan. The Institute of Medicine defines patient-centered are as "providing care that is respectful of, and responsive to, individual patient preferences, needs and values, and ensuring that patient values guide all clinical decisions."[16]

Also included in patient-centered care is the ability of patients to self-manage behavior change. Self-efficacy increases when patients are engaged in their own care.[17] MI increases patient self-efficacy while promoting patient–practitioner interactions and effectiveness, which are key factors in chronic disease management.[17] Furthermore, MI helps patients better manage chronic disease, especially those conditions that require lifestyle modification such as hypertension, heart disease, or diabetes. Studies have shown found that MI has a greater impact on lifestyle choices such as diet, exercise, and chronic disease management than typical approaches such as patient education and risk reduction interventions.[18]

A large body of evidence has been published describing the benefit of using MI across a broad range of behaviors including medication adherence.[19] In a recent meta-analysis that included randomized controlled trials that compared MI to a control group and a numerical measure of adherence, results demonstrated improved self-reported and objectives measure of adherence in the MI groups.[20] Included were trials with MI delivered by phone, face-to-face individual, face-to-face group, or mixed delivery. Studies of patients using ART were the most common, and a majority included individual face-to-face MI sessions. The results of the meta-analysis showed improved adherence in the MI groups.[20] In a second systematic review designed to assess successful adherence interventions in patients with hypertension, those interventions that included MI were more effective.[21]

MI has been shown to be beneficial in patients with diabetes mellitus. In a systematic review, included were studies in adults with type 2 diabetes where MI was included as an intervention compared to a control group of usual care. Outcomes measured were changes in health behaviors that influence diabetes and clinical outcomes. MI was effective in aspects of diabetes management that included dietary changes and modification.[18]

MI was feasible and acceptable in a resource-constrained setting in Brazil.[22] In this trial, community health agents (CHAs) conducted the MI sessions. The CHAs received 32 hours of training in MI prior to conducting the MI intervention. Specifically, the CHAs were trained to help the participants to identify their own self-management skills and goals regarding medication adherence, exercise, and diet. The CHAs continued to receive MI training through the 6-month intervention periods that consisted of monthly sessions, which were 4 hours long. Patient outcomes were measured using the Patient Assessment of Chronic Illness Care,[23] Morisky scale,[24] and the Summary of Diabetes Self-Care Activities.[25] Clinical outcomes measured included hemoglobin A1c (HbA1c), blood pressure, and lipids. Clinical measures showed slight improvement in HbA1c and significant improvement in lipids. No changes were seen in blood pressure. Patients who received home visits from the trained CHAs reported significant improvement with their satisfaction of the diabetes care they received.

Studies in patients with hypertension that included MI as a key intervention resulted in improved clinical outcomes.[26] Many of the studies focused on the adherence aspect of hypertension management.[26,27] A systematic review of interventions for adherence in patients with hypertension suggested that MI approach warranted further attention due the trends toward significance, but too few, studies in improving outcomes in patients.[21]

MI has been shown to be effective in patients with heart failure. In a study by Creber and colleagues[28] a tailored MI designed to improve self-care included patients who had a heart failure–related hospitalization and were followed after hospitalization. The results showed a trend toward significance in the MI intervention group.

MODELS FOR USING MI IN THE MANAGEMENT OF CHRONIC DISEASE: WHO PROVIDES CARE?

MI for chronic disease may be delivered by a variety of practitioners including physicians, nurse practitioners, nurses, mental health professionals, social workers, physician assistants, pharmacists, dieticians, and trained community members. MI has been effectively delivered by general practice physicians and other healthcare practitioners such as nurses and dieticians.[29,30] In addition, MI can be an effective intervention even when delivered by non-healthcare professionals.[31]

It is important to note that practitioners may undergo training while in professional educational programs, but in studies where practitioners received onsite training, clinical outcomes improved.[27] In addition, skills improved in family medicine practitioners after an 8-hour training.[32] Specifically, MI training geared toward interventions for the treatment of diabetes was feasible and successful in family medicine residents.[33]

Other work has used trained community health workers and team-based care as effective strategies[26] or other cadres of healthcare workers. A nurse-led MI as an intervention in patients with heart failure had significant improvement in heart failure self-management when compared to patients who received usual care.[28]

MI has been delivered in multiple ways including face to face, by telephone, or through mixed delivery approach. Research shows that interventions delivered over multiple days are more effective that single encounters and models that include MI across multiple clinic visits will be more successful.[21]

APPLYING MI IN PATIENTS WITH CO-MORBID MEDICAL PROBLEMS

MI can be used to help patients self-manage chronic co-morbid conditions in the context of their HIV care as well as social and cultural factors. Several studies suggest that poor control of HIV correlates with poor control of other chronic diseases such as diabetes and hypertension.[34,35] Adherence to HIV treatment may predict success managing other chronic conditions; however, patients may prioritize conditions differently according to perceived importance and level of confidence. Weiss and colleagues[36] found that adherence to ART was similar to medication adherence for co-morbid hypertension and chronic kidney disease, while Batchelder, Gonzalez, and Berg[37] found that patients were more likely to adhere to ART than diabetes medications. In both studies, patients reported that ART was more necessary than medications for other conditions, highlighting the central role of patients' medication beliefs to adherence. Adherence interventions for HIV treatment may be adapted to develop a comprehensive self-management plan encompassing co-morbid conditions.

The need to address HIV management alongside co-morbid conditions presents challenges in routine patient care. It may be difficult to devote adequate time to all chronic diseases or problems during office visits. Using the agenda mapping and prioritizing the issues that the patient needs to address would be helpful to focus the sessions. Additionally, patients may become overwhelmed or ambivalent by the need to make behavior changes to address multiple health needs. In this situation, MI puts the patient's own motivations for change at the center of the conversation while allowing the practitioner to explore barriers and management strategies with the patient. Skillful use of MI can empower patients to identify steps to manage chronic conditions in their own social and cultural context.

The following conversation illustrates how a practitioner can use MI to promote self-management integrating both HIV and medical co-morbidities.

Practitioner: Would it be alright if we spend some time now discussing your blood pressure control? (Asking permission and focusing)

Patient: Sure.

Practitioner: I remember we planned to start a new blood pressure medication last time you were here. How have you been doing with that since we last spoke? (Open-ended question)

Patient: I picked up the prescription and took it for a few days, but it made me feel "off" so I stopped taking it.

Practitioner: You believe you may have had a side effect to the medication. (Reflection) How did it make you feel? (Eliciting using open-ended question)

Patient: Well, I don't know if I had a side effect exactly, but I do start to worry about taking so many medications at once. I've heard that too many medications can be hard on the kidneys.

Practitioner: You're concerned that all these medications may be causing more harm than good. (Reflection)

Patient: Well, I take my HIV medication almost every day and that's been working for a long time, plus my other 3 pills, but eventually all those medications in my system are bound to cause some harm.

Practitioner: You are concerned about how multiple medications maybe affecting your overall health; at the same time, you have been committed to taking your HIV medications and your CD4 and viral load were where they should be the last time we checked. (Reflection)

Patient: Yes, I know how much important it is to stick to my HIV medications. I care so much about my quality of life.

Practitioner: Compared to the importance of taking HIV medications, what do you see as the benefits of keeping your blood pressure controlled? (Evocative question and focusing on eliciting change talk)

Patient: I know I need to do whatever it takes to keep my blood pressure controlled since it can help prevent heart attack and stroke, but I also eat better than most people and try to get exercise.

Practitioner: And you see the importance of eating healthy and keeping up with physical activity that will help your heart health and control your blood pressure. (Affirmation) Do you mind if I share with you some additional information about this medication and effects of blood pressure control? (Asking permission)

Patient: Okay.

Practitioner: [Discusses the protective effect of blood pressure control kidney function and low evidence of drug interactions with other medications,] So, what are your thoughts now? (Evocative question)

Patient: Well, if there are no interactions with my other medications, then I'll give it another try.

Practitioner: You are making a very important decision about how to manage your health. (Reflection/affirmation). How do you see this fitting into your current medication regimen? [Continues discussion about medication management system.] (Evocative question)

Through reflections and evocative questions, practitioners are able to explore sources of ambivalence regarding chronic disease management in the context of a patient's HIV care and guide the patient through the process of resolving it. MI encourages patients to move toward health behavior change while respecting their autonomy.

REFERENCES

1. Wandeler G, Johnson LF, Egger M. Trends in life expectancy of HIV-positive adults on antiretroviral therapy across the globe: comparisons with general population. *Curr Opin HIV AIDS*. 2016;11(5):492–500.
2. US Department of Health and Human Services. Healthy People. 2020. https://www.healthypeople.gov/.
3. Naghavi M, Wang H, Resnicow K, et al. Global, regional, and national age-sex specific all-cause and cause-specific mortality for 240 causes of death, 1990–2013: a systematic analysis for the Global Burden of Disease Study 2013. *Lancet*. 2015;385(9963):117–171.
4. Murray CJ, Vos T, Lozano R, et al. (2012). Disability-adjusted life years (DALYs) for 291 diseases and injuries in 21 regions, 1990–2010: a systematic analysis for the Global Burden of Disease Study 2010. *Lancet*. 2012;380(9859):2197–2223.
5. Greene M, Steinman MA, Mcnicholl IR, Valcour V. Polypharmacy, drug-drug interactions, and potentially inappropriate medications in older adults with human immunodeficiency virus infection. *J Am Geriatr Soc*. 2014;62(3):447–453.

6. Smit M, Brinkman K, Geerlings S, et al. Future challenges for clinical care of an ageing population infected with HIV: a modelling study. *Lancet Infect Dis.* 2015;15(7):810–818.

7. World Health Organization. "Ageing well" must be a global priority. https://www.who.int/mediacentre/news/releases/2014/lancet-ageing-series/en/. Published November 6, 2014.

8. Obel N, Thomsen HF, Kronborg G, et al. Ischemic heart disease in HIV-infected and HIV-uninfected individuals: a population-based cohort study. *Clin Infect Dis.* 2007;44(12):1625–1631.

9. Butt AA, Chang CC, Kuller L, et al. Risk of heart failure with human immunodeficiency virus in the absence of prior diagnosis of coronary heart disease. *Arch Intern Med.* 2011;171(8):737–743.

10. Brown TT, Cole SR, Li X, et al. Antiretroviral therapy and the prevalence and incidence of diabetes mellitus in the multicenter AIDS cohort study. *Arch Intern Med.* 2005;165(10):1179–1184.

11. US Department of Health and Human Services. Panel on Opportunistic Infections in HIV-infected Adults and Adolescents. https://aidsinfo.nih.gov/guidelines. Retrieved on March 12, 2019.

12. Bhavan KP, Kampalath VN, Overton ET. (2008). The aging of the HIV epidemic. *Curr HIV/AIDS Rep.* 2008;5(3):150–158.

13. Magee MJ, Narayan KM. Global confluence of infectious and non-communicable diseases: the case of type 2 diabetes. *Prev Med.* 2013;57(3):149–145.

14. Chu C, Selwyn PA. An epidemic in evolution: the need for new models of HIV care in the chronic disease era. *J Urban Health.* 2011;88(3):556–566.

15. Bygbjerg IC. Double burden of non-communicable and infectious diseases in developing countries. *Science.* 2012;337(6101):1499–1501.

16. Institute of Medicine. *Crossing the Quality Chasm: A New Health System for the 21st Century.* Washington, DC: The National Academies Press; 2001.

17. Bodenheimer T, Lorig K, Holman, H, Grumbach, K. Patient self-management of chronic disease in primary care. *JAMA.* 2002;288(19):2469–2475.

18. Ekong G, Kavookjian J. Motivational interviewing and outcomes in adults with type 2 diabetes: a systematic review. *Patient Educ Couns.* 2016;99(6):944–952.

19. Burke BL, Arkowitz H, Menchola M. The efficacy of motivational interviewing: a meta-analysis of controlled clinical trials. *J Consult Clin Psychol.* 2003;71(5):843–861.

20. Palacio A, Garay D, Langer B, Taylor J, Wood BA, Tamariz L. Motivational interviewing improves medication adherence: a systematic review and meta-analysis. *J Gen Intern Med.* 2016;31(8):929–940.

21. Conn VS, Ruppar TM, Chase JA, Enriquez M, Cooper PS. Interventions to improve medication adherence in hypertensive patients: systematic review and meta-analysis. *Curr Hypertens Rep.* 2015;17(12):94.

22. Nascimento TM, Resnicow K, Nery M, et al. A pilot study of a community health agent-led type 2 diabetes self-management program using motivational interviewing-based approaches in a public primary care center in São Paulo, Brazil. *BMC Health Serv Res.* 2017;17(1):32.

23. Glasgow RE, Whitesides H, Nelson CC, King DK. Use of the Patient Assessment of Chronic Illness Care (PACIC) with diabetic patients: relationship to patient characteristics, receipt of care, and self-management. *Diabetes Care.* 2005;28(11):2655–2661.

24. Morisky DE, Green LW, Levine DM. Concurrent and predictive validity of a self-reported measure of medication adherence. *Med Care.* 1986;24(1):67–74.

25. Toobert DJ. Glasgow RE. Assessing diabetes self-management: the summary of diabetes self-care activities questionnaire. In: Bradley C, ed. *Handbook of Psychology and Diabetes*. Chur, Switzerland: Harwood Academic, 1994: 351–375. ·

26. Kravetz JD, Walsh RF. Team-based hypertension management to improve blood pressure control. *J Prim Care Community Health*. 2016;7(4):272–275.

27. Ma C, Zhou Y, Zhou W. Huang C. Evaluation of the effect of motivational interviewing counselling on hypertension care. *Patient Educ Couns*. 2014;95:231–237.

28. Creber R, Patey M, Lee CS, Kuan A, Jurgens C, Riegel B. Motivational interviewing to improve self-care for patients with chronic heart failure: MITI-HF randomized controlled trial. *Patient Educ Couns*. 2016;99(2):256–256.

29. Stott NC, Rees M, Rollnick S, Pill RM, Hackett P. Professional responses to innovation in clinical method: diabetes care and negotiating skills. *Patient Educ Couns*. 1996;29(1):67–73.

30. Mhurchú CN, Margetts BM, Speller V. Randomized clinical trial comparing the effectiveness of two dietary interventions for patients with hyperlipidaemia. *Clin Sci*. 1998;95(4):479–487.

31. Low KG, Giasson H, Connors S, Freeman D, Weiss R. Testing the effectiveness of motivational interviewing as a weight reduction strategy for obese cardiac patients: a pilot study. *Int J Behav Med*. 2013;20(1):77–81.

32. Lazare K, Moaveni A. Introduction of a motivational interviewing curriculum for family medicine residents. *Fam Med*. 2016;48(4):305–308.

33. Nightingale B, Gopalan P, Azzam P, Douaihy A, Conti T. Teaching brief motivational interventions for diabetes to family medicine residents. *Fam Med*. 2016;48(3):187–193.

34. Davies ML, Johnson MD, Brown JN, Bryan WE, Townsend ML. Predictors of glycaemic control among HIV-positive veterans with diabetes. *Int J STD AIDS*. 2015;26(4):262–267.

35. Monroe AK, Chander G, Moore RD. Control of medical comorbidities in individuals with HIV. *J Acquir Immune Defic Syndr*. 2011;58(5):458–462.

36. Weiss JJ, Konstantinidis I, Boueilh A, et al. Illness perceptions, medication beliefs, and adherence to antiretrovirals and medications for comorbidities in adults with HIV infection and hypertension or chronic kidney disease. *J Acquir Immune Defic Syndr*. 2016;73(4):403–410.

37. Batchelder AW, Gonzalez JS, Berg KM. Differential medication nonadherence and illness beliefs in co-morbid HIV and type 2 diabetes. *J Behav Med*. 2014;37(2):266–275.

11 Substance Use and Motivational Interviewing

Liu yi Lin, Linda R. Frank, and Antoine Douaihy

The term *syndemics,* applied in the context of HIV/AIDS by Singer[1] describes an intertwined set of public health problems such as mental health, substance use/addiction, and violence/abuse that additively increase vulnerability to negative health outcomes.[2] Additionally, syndemic theory suggests that these mutually reinforcing health problems are fueled by social and economic inequities.[1,3] Substance use disorder (SUD) is a highly prevalent condition in people living with HIV (PLWH), and, together, the 2 disease processes constitute a syndemic that deleteriously impact one another.[4,5] SUD is defined by a problematic pattern of behaviors related to the use of a substance(s), with impaired control over use leading to social and role dysfunction, risky use despite physical and psychological hazards, and pharmacological dependence with tolerance and withdrawal.[6]

IMPACT OF SUBSTANCE USE ON THE HIV CONTINUUM OF CARE

Currently, an estimated 1.1 million people are infected with HIV in the United States, and only about half of PLWH are engaged in care or have achieved viral suppression.[7,8] SUD remains a main driver in the transmission of HIV in the United States and accounts for 9% of newly diagnosed HIV cases. Persons who inject drugs are at 22 times higher risk of acquiring HIV than the general population.[8,9] Importantly, SUD appears to negatively impact each stage of the HIV care continuum as studies have shown that SUD is associated with delay in diagnosis, poor engagement and retention in treatment, unsuppressed viral load, increased sexual risk behaviors, and increased burdens on health care systems.[10–12] The burden of SUD and HIV disproportionally affect vulnerable and disenfranchised populations, and factors such as trauma, poverty, and stigma continue to contribute to gaps in care.[13]

Screening for and treating substance use may contribute to closing the gaps in HIV care continuum outcomes and help achieve the UNAIDS 90-90-90 goal of 90% diagnosis, 90% antiretroviral therapy (ART) treatment, and 90% HIV viral suppression by 2020.[14] Major challenges to the UNAIDS 90-90-90 goals have been identified in the United States and abroad. For example, in Oakland, California, criminal justice involvement was associated with increased rates of HIV and hepatitis C testing but did not result in improved treatment engagement. Those who reported receiving SUD treatment, however, were more likely to engage in HIV care than those not receiving treatment.[15] Additionally, sex workers in Cambodia who used amphetamine were less likely to remain in care at 12 months.[16]

Multiple prior studies have shown high rates of SUD in PLWH and lifetime prevalence of SUD in PLWH is estimated to be 84%.[5,10,17] PLWH smoke at higher rate than the general population, and prior estimates have shown a prevalence of 40% to 70%.[18,19] Alcohol is often a significant contributor to adverse HIV outcomes: 53.4% of PLWH report current use of alcohol and rates of heavy drinking and binge drinking are higher in PLWH compared to general population.[12,20] Furthermore, PLWH who report heavy drinking experienced increased odds of failing to achieve sustained HIV viral suppression.[21] Use of stimulants such as cocaine and amphetamines is also common and have a prevalence rate of 11% and 13%, respectively, among PLWH.[5] Similar to alcohol, use of stimulants such as with methylenedioxymethamphetamine can cause sexual disinhibition and high-risk sexual behavior, furthering the risk of HIV transmission.

Opioid use is also more prevalent among PLWH than general population, and estimates ranges from 4% to 9%.[5,22] The recent opioid epidemic has been linked with outbreak of HIV in rural populations such as in Austin, Indiana, due to syringe-sharing among people who were injecting prescription oxymorphone.[23] This last example illustrates the syndemic nature of HIV and SUD and the importance of addressing both conditions in an integrated and MI-based approach addressing both behaviors related to self-management of HIV and substance use.

CHALLENGES IN THE TREATMENT OF PEOPLE WITH CO-OCCURRING HIV AND SUD

Multiple behavioral, structural, and environmental factors contribute to the unique challenge of caring for patients with SUD and HIV. Substance use functions as a direct and indirect vector for HIV transmission in that IV injection of drugs facilitate virus infection by sharing of injection equipment, and the effects of certain drugs can lead to disinhibition for increased risky sexual behaviors.[10,24] Additionally, patients who have the "triple diagnosis" of HIV, SUD, and a co-morbid psychiatric illness account for 10% to 25% of PLWH.[10] This highly at-risk population faces complex health and socioeconomic needs, significant stigma, and lack of access to care. Not only are they more likely to experience poverty, homelessness, unemployment, violence, and trauma, but they may also face other barriers such as incarceration and discrimination from healthcare practitioners.[7,9] Prior studies have shown that "triple diagnosis" is associated with delayed HIV diagnosis, suboptimal engagement in treatment, reduced likelihood of being prescribed ART, and medication nonadherence.[4,10,25] Furthermore, people with a co-occurring SUD and HIV are more likely to be hospitalized for HIV-related symptoms and have a higher morbidity and mortality compared to those who do not use substances.[26,27] Thus, practitioners caring for this vulnerable population should utilize a patient-centered and motivational approach to increase patient's self-efficacy and engagement in treatment.[24,28]

ROLE OF MOTIVATIONAL INTERVIEWING IN THE TREATMENT OF PATIENTS WITH CO-OCCURRING HIV AND A SUD

For patients living with both HIV and a SUD, a comprehensive approach to care must include 3 goals as outlined by Substance Abuse and Mental Health Services Administration: (i) living substance free and sober, (ii) slowing the progression of HIV/AIDS, and (iii) reducing HIV risk-taking.[29] To accomplish these goals, practitioners can optimize care with a patient-centered approach that encourages treatment engagement and collaborative goal-setting along with identifying systems issues that can interfere with the HIV care continuum for this population. Furthermore, addressing service agency stigma can facilitate engagement in treatment.[30]

Integrated HIV care is defined as a model in which specialists from multiple disciplines collaborate to provide PLWH with onsite primary care, HIV specialty services, and other services such as treatment for hepatitis C, psychiatric and substance use, and social and peer support services. HIV and mental health/substance use services can be integrated within a single facility or multifacility or through coordinated care by nonphysician case managers.[31] Patients involved in HIV-integrated care were more likely to achieve viral suppression on ART.[32] Moreover, existing evidence suggest that this integrated HIV and mental health model may be linked to improved patient and service delivery outcomes in diverse settings.[31] MI can be utilized across all components of integrated care as a clinical style or as an approach to address behavior change (Figure 11.1). MI can serve as a powerful tool to help engage, treat, and retain PLWH using drugs and alcohol to improve their HIV continuum of care and help them address their substance use and other related behaviors. For example, Project HOPE, a National Institute on Drug Abuse Clinical Trials Network study used peer navigators trained in MI to link hospitalized patients with untreated HIV and SUDs to HIV treatment.[33] In that study, providing monetary incentives (contingency management) to attend peer navigator sessions increased visit attendance and HIV viral suppression at 6 months.[34]

The first stage of the HIV care continuum is the testing and diagnosis of HIV. MI has been shown to be effective in encouraging high-risk patient populations to receive testing and a recent systemic review of MI shows promise in increasing health screening uptake.[35,36] Additionally, given that HIV remains frequently underdiagnosed among patients with SUD, testing should be offered in substance use treatment facilities, correctional facilities, and emergency rooms where there is a high prevalence of patients with SUD.[24]

Once a patient is diagnosed with HIV, the next step in the HIV care continuum is prompt linkage to care. In 2016, only 3 out of 4 persons receiving the diagnosis of HIV were linked to care within 1 month.[7] Multitudes of barriers have consistently been identified as risk factors: poverty, housing insecurity, lack of insurance or access to primary care prior to HIV diagnosis, SUDs, and psychiatric disorder.[37] MI can be utilized in a strength-based case management model to identify a patient's strengths and skills

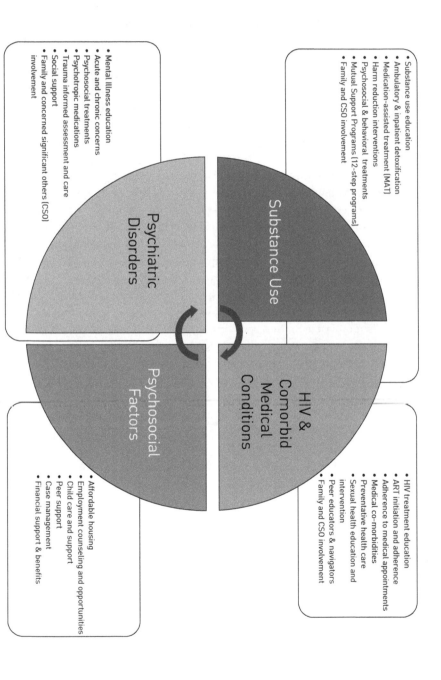

- Substance use education
- Ambulatory & inpatient detoxification
- Medication-assisted treatment (MAT)
- Harm reduction interventions
- Psychosocial & behavioral treatments
- Mutual Support Programs (12-step programs)
- Family and CSO involvement

- Mental Illness education
- Acute and chronic concerns
- Psychosocial treatments
- Psychotropic medications
- Trauma informed assessment and care
- Social support
- Family and concerned significant others (CSO) involvement

Substance Use

Psychiatric Disorders

HIV & Comorbid Medical Conditions

Psychosocial Factors

- HIV treatment education
- ART initiation and adherence
- Adherence to medical appointments
- Medical co-morbidities
- Preventative health care
- Sexual health education and intervention
- Peer educators & navigators
- Family and CSO involvement

- Affordable housing
- Employment counseling and opportunities
- Child care and support
- Peer support
- Case management
- Financial support & benefits

FIGURE 11.1. Integrated care model: applications of MI across all components. SO = concerned significant others. ART = antiretroviral therapy.

to attain needed resources. This brief intervention has shown significantly higher rates of receiving HIV care than the standard care group.[38]

The next stage in the HIV care continuum is engagement in care and prescription of HIV ART treatment. As with each prior step of care, there is increasing dropout and lost to care of patients at each subsequent stage. Based on the most recent data from 2015, it is estimated at that only 63% of PLWH have received care, and only 49% are engaged in care.[7] It is critical at this stage of the treatment intervention process to address both HIV and SUD in an integrated approach, as relapses in using substances frequently lead to nonadherence with ART. The traditional model of "abstinence-only" approach is effective for a small portion of patients. Healthcare practitioners should be cognizant that patients frequently use substances to manage their own mood or self-medicate. Although these behaviors may be unhealthy, it is difficult for patients to break this cycle of substance use without first addressing the role that the substance currently plays their lives.[29] MI is well-suited for exploration of these psychosocial factors and ambivalence to change and seeks to develop discrepancy between a patients' present behavior and their goals and value system. By addressing ambivalence and drawing from a patient's own resources, MI engages patient to actively problem-solve and interrupt self-destructive cycles of behaviors.

The final component of the HIV care continuum is patient retention in care and HIV viral suppression. Currently, it is estimated that only 30% of PLWH have achieved viral suppression.[7] Lack of attendance at regularly scheduled appointment and nonadherence to ART is associated with worse clinical outcomes and further contribute to ongoing HIV transmission to others.[39] MI can be utilized at this stage to promote and reinforce ART adherence.[40] Additionally, clinicians should also use MI to counsel patients on risk-reduction behaviors including avoidance of sharing needles and equipment for drug injection and using condoms with sexual activities. By reinforcing patient's intrinsic motivation to adhere to medications and reduce risky behaviors, practitioners can support patients' self-efficacy and improve both physical and mental health.

CASE EXAMPLE

The patient is a 27-year-old man who has a history of opioid use disorder and alcohol use disorder. He first starting using alcohol at age 12 with a history of binge drinking and "blacking out" on weekends. He became addicted to opioid pills after an injury in his teenage years and transitioned to using heroin intravenously in the last 2 years. He is alienated from his family due to his addiction, and he is currently homeless and stays in various shelters around the city. He was diagnosed with HIV 1 year ago when he was hospitalized for pneumonia, and he has been referred to the local HIV clinic. However, he has only intermittently followed up with care and has admitted to intermittent adherence to ART. This MI conversation addresses his struggles with adhering to ART and its connection to his substance use:

Practitioner: How have been you been doing with taking your HIV medications? (Open question)

Patient: I have been doing okay, I guess. I miss a dose here or there. I don't see what the problem is, though—I have been feeling fine lately.

Practitioner: You feel that your HIV illness cannot be much affected if you haven't felt sick. (Complex reflection)

Patient: Well, not really. I mean, I know that I should keep on top of the medications, ... but it has been difficult to leave the shelter because of the weather, and I have to walk to the pharmacy to get the medications.

Practitioners: You have had difficulty picking up the medications, and at the same time you know that you have to take them consistently and every day. What are your thoughts regarding how you would like to address this? (Reflection followed by open-ended question)

Patient: I don't know, I guess I can get a ride from someone at the shelter. I don't want people to know about my HIV though . . .

Practitioner: You are scared that people might know about your HIV status, judge you, or even possibly threaten you. (Complex reflection)

Patient: Exactly, I feel like that I have to hide it, and I don't want people to know that I am sick.

Practitioner: You want to stay healthy and for people to think that about you too. What do you think will be important for you to do to achieve that? (Complex reflection and eliciting change talk and personal goals)

Patient: I guess I have to take my medications regularly and not miss even one time and follow up with my doctors. I definitely don't want to go back to the hospital again.

Practitioner: You clearly know what matters to you, and you know what works for you to control your HIV illness. How confident are that you can follow through with sticking to your medications and attending with your clinic appointments, on a scale to 10, 1 not confident and 10 extremely confident? (Affirmation/complex reflection followed by confidence ruler).

Patient: I would say 6, I know I need to do it, but I struggle with not having a stable place to live with limited support. My family refuses to talk with me, and I ended using heroin and alcohol sometimes to deal with these issues.

Practitioner: You have been struggling with so many issues that make it hard for you to prioritize taking your medications regularly and making it to your appointments. I appreciate your making the effort and coming to the clinic today despite your limited resources and the challenges you are facing. What puts you at 6, not a 3? (Complex reflection followed by an affirmation and then confidence ruler)

Patient: Thanks for working with me. Well, I believe I can do it because I was able to do it before, taking my medications consistently and sticking to my appointments and even not using alcohol or heroin for some time.

Practitioner: You have a good experience with making changes in the past and you believe you can try again to make sure you stay healthy. How do you feel about discussing some potential resources we can offer you here to make it easier for you to take medications and stick to treatment and get your life back on track? (Complex reflection followed by evocative question)

Patient: Sure.

Practitioner: Yes, of course, we can review the options. First, is it okay with you to discuss your substance use and how it has been affecting you? (Asking permission)

Patient: Yes, sure. It has been more of a problem recently—I mean I am homeless now, I have no job, and my heroin and alcohol use are getting out of control.

Practitioner: You are concerned about your heroin and alcohol use and their impacts on your life, that you have seen falling apart recently. (Complex reflection)

Patient: Yes, totally. I need to get back into treatment for my drug addictions, I know I can stop using, but I can't do it on my own. I need help.

Practitioner: You have seen the painful impact of your use of heroin and alcohol on your adherence to medications and clinic visits, and you have experienced how your life fell apart as a result of your use and particularly losing your family. Now you are determined to control your addiction and get your life back on track. How do you feel about exploring some treatment options for your addiction to heroin and alcohol? (Summary statement followed by a complex reflection and open question)

Patient: Yes, definitely.

Practitioner: So, we have medication options in the clinic such as buprenorphine or naltrexone injection, and we can refer you to our therapist in the clinic for counseling, or we can consider referring you to our addiction treatment program for a comprehensive treatment including counseling and seeing a psychiatrist. Another option we can consider is a residential treatment program for a short period of time and then connecting you with our addiction treatment program after you complete the residential program. Of course, we will continue working with you here to manage your HIV. Another resource we can offer is our peer support program to help with resources in the community and housing. (Menu of options and resources)

Patient: Wow, you have so much to offer. That is confusing a bit. Can you tell me more about the peer support person?

Practitioner: Yes, I must have overwhelmed you with all these options. We can definitely review them again, and you can decide what would be the best option for you, and we can facilitate the process. So, yes, the peer support person is an individual with lived experience, meaning who struggled with HIV and even substance use and can support you and help you navigate the system of care and find resources in the community. What do you think? (Complex reflection/giving information)

Patient: Yes, that would be a great resource. Can we start with connecting me with that person and I can think more about all the options you mentioned? I've heard of buprenorphine. I may want to try it.

Practitioner: Okay sure will do.

This clinical case is a demonstration of how MI attends to multiple intersecting behaviors which demonstrates how HIV infection and substance use are so intertwined. It also demonstrates how to facilitate behavior changes for PLWH struggling with a co-occurring SUD.

Addressing gaps in the HIV care continuum in persons with a SUD and HIV is an ongoing and considerable challenge that requires a comprehensive and an integrated approach that targets all components, settings, and health practitioners involved in the HIV care continuum for the patient. Developing, testing, and implementing new interventions targeting PLWH and SUD are clearly needed. MI is well-positioned to influence and achieve positive change in behaviors within HIV care, substance use, and integrated care systems.

REFERENCES

1. Singer M. AIDS and the health crisis of the U.S. urban poor: the perspective of critical medical anthropology. *Soc Sci Med.* 1994;39(7):931–948.
2. Singer MC, Erickson PI, Badiane L, et al. Syndemics, sex and the city: understanding sexually transmitted diseases in social and cultural context. *Soc Sci Med.* 2006;63(8):2010–2021.
3. Singer M, Clair S. Syndemics and public health: reconceptualizing disease in bio-social context. *Med Anthropol Q.* 2003;17(4):423–441.
4. Altice FL, Kamarulzaman A, Soriano VV, Schechter M, Friedland GH. Treatment of medical, psychiatric, and substance-use comorbidities in people infected with HIV who use drugs. *Lancet.* 2010;376(9738):367–387.
5. Hartzler B, Dombrowski JC, Crane HM, et al. Prevalence and predictors of substance use disorders among HIV care enrollees in the United States. *AIDS Behav.* 2017;21(4):1138–1148.
6. American Psychiatric Association. *Diagnostic and Statistical Manual of Mental Disorders.* 5th ed. Washington, DC: American Psychiatric Association; 2013.
7. Centers for Disease Control and Prevention. HIV and substance use in the United States. https://www.cdc.gov/hiv/risk/substanceuse.html. Last updated September 21, 2018.
8. Hess K, Johnson A, S Hu, X Li, et al. Diagnoses of HIV Infection in the United States and Dependent Areas. *HIV Surveillance Report.* 2016;2(28). https://www.cdc.gov/hiv/pdf/library/reports/surveillance/cdc-hiv-surveillance-report-2016-vol-28.pdf.
9. AVERT. People who inject drugs, HIV and AIDS. https://www.avert.org/professionals/hiv-social-issues/key-affected-populations/people-inject-drugs. Last updated February 15, 2019.
10. Durvasula R, Miller TR. Substance abuse treatment in persons with HIV/AIDS: challenges in managing triple diagnosis. *Behav Med.* 2014;40(2):43–52.
11. Gwadz M, De Guzman R, Freeman R, et al. Exploring how substance use impedes engagement along the HIV care continuum: a qualitative study. *Front Public Health.* 2016;4:62.
12. Vagenas P, Azar MM, Copenhaver MM, Springer SA, Molina PE, Altice FL. The impact of alcohol use and related disorders on the HIV continuum of care: a systematic review: alcohol and the HIV continuum of care. *Curr HIV/AIDS Rep.* 2015;12(4):421–436.
13. Pellowski JA, Kalichman SC, Matthews KA, Adler N. A pandemic of the poor: social disadvantage and the U.S. HIV epidemic. *Am Psychol.* 2013;68(4):197–209.
14. UNAIDS, Joint United Nations Programme on HIV/AIDS. 90-90-90: an ambitious treatment target to help end the AIDS epidemic. http://www.unaids.org/sites/default/files/media_asset/90-90-90_en_0.pdf. Published October 2014.
15. Lambdin BH, Kral AH, Comfort M, Lopez AM, Lorvick J. Associations of criminal justice and substance use treatment involvement with HIV/HCV testing and the HIV treatment cascade among people who use drugs in Oakland, California. *Addict Sci Clin Pract.* 2017;12(1):13.
16. Muth S, Len A, Evans JL, et al. HIV treatment cascade among female entertainment and sex workers in Cambodia: impact of amphetamine use and an HIV prevention program. *Addict Sci Clin Pract.* 2017;12(1):20.
17. Bing EG, Burnam MA, Longshore D, et al. Psychiatric disorders and drug use among human immunodeficiency virus-infected adults in the United States. *Arch Gen Psychiatry.* 2001;58(8):721–728.
18. Calvo M, Laguno M, Martínez M, Martínez E. Effects of tobacco smoking on HIV-infected individuals. *AIDS Rev.* 2015;17(1):47–55.

19. Mdodo R, Frazier EL, Dube SR, et al. Cigarette smoking prevalence among adults with HIV compared with the general adult population in the United States: cross-sectional surveys. *Ann Intern Med.* 2015;162(5):335–344.

20. Molina PE, Bagby GJ, Nelson S. Biomedical consequences of alcohol use disorders in the HIV-infected host. *Curr HIV Res.* 2014;12(4):265–275.

21. Cook RL, Zhou Z, Kelso-Chichetto NE, et al. Alcohol consumption patterns and HIV viral suppression among persons receiving HIV care in Florida: an observational study. *Addict Sci Clin Pract.* 2017;12(1):22. doi:10.1186/s13722-017-0090-0

22. Broz D, Wejnert C, Pham HT, et al. HIV infection and risk, prevention, and testing behaviors among injecting drug users: National HIV Behavioral Surveillance System, 20 U.S. cities, 2009. *MMWR Surveill Summ.* 2014;63(6):1–51.

23. Conrad C, Bradley HM, Broz D, et al. Community outbreak of HIV infection linked to injection drug use of oxymorphone—Indiana, 2015. *MMWR.* 2015;64(16):443–444.

24. Amin P, Douaihy A. Substance use disorders in people living with human immunodeficiency virus/AIDS. *Nurs Clin North Am.* 2018;53(1):57–65.

25. Friedland, G. HIV therapy in "triple-diagnosed" patients: HIV infection, drug use, and mental illness. http://hivinsite.ucsf.edu/InSite?page=md-rr-05. Published May 15, 2001. Updated January 2002.

26. Croxford S, Kitching A, Desai S, et al. Mortality and causes of death in people diagnosed with HIV in the era of highly active antiretroviral therapy compared with the general population: an analysis of a national observational cohort. *Lancet Public Health.* 2017;2(1):e35–e46.

27. Delorenze GN, Weisner C, Tsai AL, Satre DD, Quesenberry CP. Excess mortality among HIV-infected patients diagnosed with substance use dependence or abuse receiving care in a fully integrated medical care program. *Alcohol Clin Exp Res.* 2011;35(2):203–210.

28. Johnson MO, Neilands TB, Dilworth SE, Morin SF, Remien RH, Chesney MA. The role of self-efficacy in HIV treatment adherence: validation of the HIV Treatment Adherence Self-Efficacy Scale (HIV-ASES). *J Behav Med.* 2008;30(5):359–370.

29. Substance Abuse and Mental Health Services Administration. Treatment for persons with HIV/AIDS. Treatment Improvement Protocol (TIP) No. 37. https://store.samhsa.gov/system/files/sma12-4137.pdf. First published 2000. Updated 2014.

30. Grau LE, Griffiths-Kundishora A, Heimer R. Barriers and facilitators of the HIV care continuum in Southern New England for people with drug or alcohol use and living with HIV/AIDS: perspectives of HIV surveillance experts and service providers. *Addict Sci Clin Pract.* 2017;12(1):24.

31. Chuah FLH, Haldane VE, Cervero-liceras F, et al. Interventions and approaches to integrating HIV and mental health services: a systematic review. *Health Policy Plan.* 2017;32(Suppl 4):iv27–iv47.

32. Hoang T, Goetz MB, Yano EM, et al. The impact of integrated HIV care on patient health outcomes. *Med Care.* 2009;47(5):560–567.

33. Metsch LR, Feaster DJ, Gooden L, et al. Effect of patient navigation with or without financial incentives on viral suppression among hospitalized patients with HIV infection and substance use: a randomized clinical trial. *JAMA.* 2016;316(2):156–170.

34. Stitzer M, Matheson T, Cunningham C, et al. Enhancing patient navigation to improve intervention session attendance and viral load suppression of persons with HIV and substance use: a secondary post hoc analysis of the Project HOPE study. *Addict Sci Clin Pract.* 2017;12(1):16.

35. Miller SJ, Foran-Tuller K, Ledergerber J, Jandorf L. Motivational interviewing to improve health screening uptake: a systematic review. *Patient Educ Couns.* 2017;100(2):190–198.

36. Outlaw AY, Naar-king S, Parsons JT, Green-jones M, Janisse H, Secord E. Using motivational interviewing in HIV field outreach with young African American men who have sex with men: a randomized clinical trial. *Am J Public Health*. 2010;100(Suppl 1):S146–S151.

37. Dombrowski JC, Kent JB, Buskin SE, Stekler JD, Golden MR. Population-based metrics for the timing of HIV diagnosis, engagement in HIV care, and virologic suppression. *AIDS*. 2012;26(1):77–86.

38. Craw JA, Gardner LI, Marks G, et al. Brief strengths-based case management promotes entry into HIV medical care: results of the antiretroviral treatment access study-II. *J Acquir Immune Defic Syndr*. 2008;47(5):597–606.

39. Gardner EM, Mclees MP, Steiner JF, Del rio C, Burman WJ. The spectrum of engagement in HIV care and its relevance to test-and-treat strategies for prevention of HIV infection. *Clin Infect Dis*. 2011;52(6):793–800.

40. Palacio A, Garay D, Langer B, Taylor J, Wood BA, Tamariz L. Motivational interviewing improves medication adherence: a systematic review and meta-analysis. *J Gen Intern Med*. 2016;31(8):929–940.

12 Emotional Management, Psychological Issues, and Motivational Interviewing

Pierre N. Azzam

CLINICAL CASE: PART 1

A 52-year old man with HIV, recurrent major depression, and remitted alcohol use disorder is seen in the infectious diseases (ID) clinic for routine care and antiretroviral medication maintenance. The patient was diagnosed with HIV infection 9 years ago, after a sexual contact while intoxicated. At the time of HIV exposure, the patient was in the midst of a depressive episode and had been terminated from his long-time employment as a carpenter at a local construction company. The patient had missed several work days due to anergia and then lost his carpentry license after presenting to the jobsite under the influence of alcohol. The patient has since maintained odd jobs and found himself isolated within his community and ostracized by his family for being HIV-positive. He presents to the ID clinic for follow-up evaluation 3 weeks after serum laboratory values demonstrated a sharp decline in CD4 count and rise in viral load from the prior 6-month test results.

EMOTIONAL DISTRESS IMPACTING PEOPLE LIVING WITH HIV

The rise in global disease burden associated with depression, anxiety, and stress-related conditions underscores the value of readily available and highly efficient mental health interventions; this is particularly compelling in the care of people living with HIV (PLWH). Depressive disorders are believed to affect between 20% and 40% of PLWH[1,2] and negatively impact functional health status and antiretroviral medication adherence and contributes to the advancement of HIV-associated disease.[3–5] Albeit less-well elucidated, anxiety and stress-related conditions are also commonly co-morbid with HIV infection and exacerbate disease markers and subjective indices of discomfort.[6–8] The progression of HIV infection and HIV-associated stigma are, themselves, correlated with a greater severity of depressive symptoms and emotional distress,[9,10] perpetuating a loop of experiences that threatens quality of life for PLWH.

The therapeutic reach of motivational interviewing (MI) has expanded, from facilitating change in substance use disorders, to enhancing therapeutic alliance and mitigating functionally impairing symptoms across psychiatric and medical conditions. In addition to targeting emotional distress and its impact on HIV disease progression, MI may be used to enhance medication adherence, reduce risky behaviors, and promote abstinence from substance use, all of which may secondarily improve emotional wellness.[11] Given the relative ease with which it can be implemented across settings, MI serves as a highly efficient tool for targeting emotional distress in PLWH.

CLINICAL CASE: PART 2

During his follow-up visit, the patient describes having experienced intermittent panic symptoms with palpitations and shortness of breath. Although he cannot identify episodic triggers, he noticed that these episodes started around the 10-year anniversary of the day he lost his carpentry license. The episodes have led the patient to experience cravings for alcohol, and although he has maintained sobriety, he feels dysphoric and disheartened by the possibility of HIV disease progression. Historically, the patient has taken an active role in his own health and well-being and would typically have asked about methods to reduce his risk for disease progression and expressed concerns about onward HIV transmission. He now appears sullen, quiet, and defeated; he avoids eye contact and asks the physician if he should be concerned about his treatment in the ID clinic since he has not been adherent to treatment.

APPROACH TO MI IN EMOTIONAL DISTRESS

The value of MI for identifying and managing emotional distress is multifaceted. Individual approaches to tailoring MI for this use have frequently referenced the relational "spirit" (e.g., collaboration) and technical skills (e.g., change reinforcement) components described by Miller and Rose.[12] In the care of individuals with depressive, anxiety, and stress-related conditions, the relational spirit of MI for promoting collaboration between patients and practitioners is particularly salient.[13] The use of MI has been shown to improve perceptions of provider empathy and communication across various settings.[14,15] Its central tenet of rapport building—using open-ended questions, affirmations, reflections, and summary statements (OARS)—allows patients who may otherwise feel stigmatized by their disease processes to gain greater comfort in disclosing psychiatric symptoms.[16]

Framing a patient's awareness of the impact of particular behaviors (e.g., physical activity, medication adherence) on subsequent emotional symptoms (e.g., energy, mood) further evokes the development of change talk and an action plan to mitigate emotional distress.[16] When engaging individuals with depression or anxiety, specific objectives for behavioral change may not be as readily apparent or as clearly delineated as in more traditional uses of MI.[17] At the same time, initial efforts to build rapport often provide subsequent insights to opportunities for change related to more subtle or covert self-limiting behaviors; these may include choices related to anergia, social withdrawal, nutrition, and interpersonal relationships.[17] In addition, using the spirit of

MI to enhance therapeutic engagement and the technical components to evoke change may naturally complement other psychotherapeutic or pharmacologic modalities that target distressing affective, behavioral, and cognitive experiences.

CLINICAL CASE: PART 3

In discussing the patient's emotional distress, the ID physician uses the MI approach. She engages the patient by reflecting on his concern about his treatment in the clinic. Rather than making premature assumptions that guide the physician to incorrect conclusions or overstating the patient's distress in a manner that places him on the defensive, the physician states: "You're a bit worried that you won't be allowed to continue your care here." The patient, feeling less guarded, explains that he blames himself for having forgotten intermittently to take his antiretroviral and antidepressant medicines over the last 3 months. The physician avoids asking closed-ended questions about patterns of medication use or responding with moralizing statements about nonadherence.

MI-ASSOCIATED OUTCOMES IN DEPRESSION, ANXIETY, AND TRAUMA-BASED DISORDERS

The value of applying MI to the care of individuals with depression has been assessed across various clinical settings, modes of delivery, and patient populations. In the primary care setting, implementing MI-based engagement with depressed individuals led to more frequent use of change talk related to mood and physical activity after as few as 4 visits.[16] Several studies in which MI was used to target behavioral changes among adolescents and young adults with conditions that are frequently co-morbid with depression—such as weight loss in obesity, glycemic control in diabetes, or breathing quality in asthma—also demonstrated secondary improvements to depressive symptoms, positive well-being, or health-related quality of life.[18-20] Challenges to in-person engagement may not limit the therapeutic reach of MI. Telephone-delivered motivational interventions have been shown to reduce depressive symptoms among individuals with various chronic disease processes, including diabetes,[21] multiple sclerosis,[22,23] traumatic brain injury,[24] and cardiovascular disease.[25,26]

In the management of anxiety- and trauma-based disorders, a small but growing body of evidence has underscored the value of MI for augmenting other action-oriented psychotherapeutic modalities, principally cognitive-behavioral therapy (CBT). In 2009, Westra and colleagues[27] demonstrated significant reductions to indices of worry and greater adherence to CBT homework in individuals with generalized anxiety disorder who engaged in four 1-hour MI-based weekly sessions in advance of CBT.[27] In a small group of individuals with social anxiety, a 3-session motivational-enhancement therapy increased patients' attendance to individual CBT sessions and their willingness to engage in contact with a therapist.[28] A 2018 meta-analysis of individuals with various anxiety, trauma-based, and obsessive-compulsive disorders further highlighted the supportive role of MI alongside CBT for reducing distressing anxiety symptoms.[29]

CLINICAL CASE: PART 4

The physician uses mirroring to summarize the patient's concerns, and soon the patient acknowledges that a recent decline in his mood, energy, and concentration has led to intermittent forgetfulness. The patient describes fear of experiencing a depressive episode as severe as the one from 10 years ago, when he last used alcohol and contracted HIV. The patient expresses a sense of guilt about not taking his medications regularly and admits that his cravings for alcohol have nearly led to another lapse. After acknowledging these challenges, the physician allows time to affirm the patient's sobriety despite intense urges and his long-standing commitment to care in the ID clinic. The patient appears less distraught. He acknowledges feeling more introspective about the anniversary of his HIV diagnosis.

MI-ASSOCIATED OUTCOMES FOR EMOTIONAL DISTRESS IN PLWH

In the care of PLWH, MI may be used to facilitate positive change in various domains, including mitigating substance use, improving nutrition and exercise, encouraging healthy sexual practices, and enhancing medication adherence.[30-32] Although relatively few in number, studies to elucidate the effects of MI on depressive and anxiety symptoms among PLWH are promising. In the specialty clinic setting, adolescents living with HIV who engaged in MI targeting safer sex practices and medication adherence also described improvements to self-efficacy and depressive indicators after 1 to 4 clinic visits.[33] Among adolescents, the developmental tension of autonomy-seeking and authority-challenging often compete with clinical recommendations for healthy behaviors, making the collaborative and nonthreatening approach of MI particularly suitable.[34] Motivational interventions have proven to be valuable on the other end of the age spectrum as well. Six months after engaging in either 1- or 4 sessions of telephone-delivered MI that focused on reducing risky sexual practices, older PLWH reported significantly lower indices of depression and anxiety.[35] When motivational language is incorporated into the holistic discussion of healthy decision-making—encouraging supportive relationships, maintaining healthcare adherence, engaging in healthy sexual practices, improving sleep hygiene, increasing healthy physical activity, and reducing substance use—the potential of MI to reduce psychiatric symptoms may be further magnified.

CLINICAL CASE: PART 5

The physician affirms the patient's decision to come to the ID clinic for a follow-up today while also experiencing lower energy and motivation. The patient expresses gratitude to the staff for providing support and describes wanting to "get on top of this depression." The physician confirms the clinic's continued commitment to the patient's care and asks about ways in which the patient and his healthcare practitioners can collaborate to "get on top of this depression together." The patient describes a desire to re-engage in counseling services through the ID clinic and motivation to use a pillbox to improve the regularity with which he remembers to take his antiretroviral and antidepressant medication. The patient schedules his next appointment in the clinic as well as a counseling session as the two develop a plan for interim telephone check-ins.

FUTURE DIRECTIONS

Either independently or in concert with other psychotherapeutic modalities, motivational interventions based on MI have proven to be valuable in the care of individuals with depressive, anxiety, and trauma-based disorders. Further studies are needed to elucidate the efficacy, advantages, and potential limitations of MI for mitigating emotional distress specifically in PLWH. Future directions for such investigations include determining the setting(s) in which MI may be most effective for PLWH (e.g., specialty ID clinic, primary care, mental health office), elucidating the acceptable modes of delivery (e.g., in-person, telephone) and their relative advantages and challenges, and establishing models for incorporating MI across various levels of supportive and clinical practice (e.g., social work, ID physicians, nurses, case managers, mental health practitioners) in a multidisciplinary HIV clinic.

REFERENCES

1. Asch SM, Kilbourne AM, Gifford AL, et al. Underdiagnosis of depression in HIV: who are we missing? *J Gen Intern Med*. 2003;18:450–460.
2. Morrison MF, Petitto JM, Ten Have T, et al. Depression and anxiety disorders in women with HIV infection. *Am J Psychiatry*. 2002;159:789–796.
3. Abas M, Ali GC, Nakimuli-Mpungu E, Chibanda D. Depression in people living with HIV in sub-Saharan Africa: time to act. *Trop Med Int Health*. 2014;19:1392–1396.
4. Yu Y, Luo D, Chen X, et al. Medication adherence to antiretroviral therapy among newly treated people with HIV. *BMC Public Health*. 2018;18:825.
5. Uthman OA, Magidson JF, Safren SA, Nachega JB. Depression and adherence to antiretroviral therapy in low-, middle-, and high-income countries: a systematic review and meta-analysis. *Curr HIV/AIDS Rep*. 2014;11:291–307.
6. Martinez A, Israelski D, Walker C, et al. Posttraumatic stress disorder in women attending human immunodeficiency virus outpatient clinics. *AIDS Patient Care STDS*. 2002;16:283–291.
7. Tsao JC, Dobalian A, Naliboff BD. Panic disorder and pain in a national sample of persons living with HIV. *Pain*. 2004;109:172–180.
8. Leserman J, Barroso J, Pence BV, et al. Trauma, stressful life events and depression predict HIV-related fatigue. *AIDS Care*. 2008;20:1258–1265.
9. Lyketsos CG, Hoover DR, Guccione M, et al. Changes in depressive symptoms as AIDS develops. *Am J Psychiatry*. 1996;153:1430–1437.
10. Rueda S, Mitra S, Chen S, et al. Examining the associations between HIV-related stigma and health outcomes in people living with HIV/AIDS: a series of meta-analyses. *BMJ Open*. 2016;6:e011453.
11. Rubak S, Sanbaek A, Lauritzien T, Christiansen B. Motivational interviewing: a systematic review and meta-analysis. *Br J Gen Pract*. 2005;55:3005–3012.
12. Miller WR, Rose GS. Toward a theory of motivational interviewing. *Am Psychol*. 2009;64:527–537.
13. Rollnick S, Miller WR. What is motivational interviewing? *Behavioural and Cognitive Psychotherapy*. 1995;23:325–334.

14. Wagoner ST, Kavookjian J. The influence of motivational interviewing on patients with inflammatory bowel disease: a systematic review of the literature. *J Clin Med Res.* 2017;9:659–666.

15. Cheret A, Durier C, Noel N, et al. Motivational interviewing training for medical students: a pilot pre-post feasibility study. *Patient Educ Couns.* 2018;101(11):1934–1941. doi:10.1016/j.pec.2018.06.011

16. Keeley RD, Burke BL, Brody D, et al. Training to use motivational interviewing techniques for depression: a cluster randomized trial. *J Am Board Fam Med.* 2014;27:621–636.

17. Westra HA, Aviram A, Doell FK. Extending motivational interviewing to the treatment of major mental health problems: current directions and evidence. *Canadian J Psychiatry.* 2011;56:643–650.

18. Freira S, Lemos MS, Williams G, et al. Effect of motivational interviewing on depression scale scores of individuals with obesity and overweight. *Psychiatry Res.* 2017;252:340–345.

19. Riekert KA, Borrelli B, Bilderback A, Rand CS. The development of a motivational interviewing intervention to promote medication adherence among inner-city, African-American adolescents with asthma. *Patient Educ Couns.* 2011;82:117–122.

20. Channon SJ, Huws-Thomas MV, Rollnick S, et al. A multicenter randomized controlled trial of motivational interviewing in teenagers with diabetes. *Diabetes Care.* 2007;30:1390–1395.

21. Dobler A, Hebeck Belnap B, et al. Telephone-delivered lifestyle support with action planning and motivational interviewing techniques to improve rehabilitation outcomes. *Rehabil Psychol.* 2018;63:170–181.

22. Turner AP, Hartoonian N, Sloan AP, et al. Improving fatigue and depression in individuals with multiple sclerosis using telephone-administered physical activity counseling. *J Consult Clin Psychol.* 2016;84:297–309.

23. Kratz AL, Ehde DM, Bombardier CH. Affective mediators of a physical activity intervention for depression in multiple sclerosis. *Rehabil Psychol.* 2014;59:57–67.

24. Bombardier CH, Bell KR, Temkin NR, et al. The efficacy of a scheduled telephone intervention for ameliorating depressive symptoms during the first year after traumatic brain injury. *J Head Trauma Rehabil.* 2009;24:230–238.

25. Tan MP, Morgan K. Psychological interventions in cardiovascular disease: an update. *Curr Opin Psychiatry.* 2015;28:371–377.

26. Lee WW, Choi KC, Yum RW, Yu DS, Chair SY. Effectiveness of motivational interviewing on lifestyle modification and health outcomes of clients at risk or diagnosed with cardiovascular diseases: a systematic review. *Int J Nurs Stud.* 2016;53:331–341.

27. Westra HA, Arkowitz H, Dozois DJA. Adding a motivational interviewing pretreatment to cognitive behavioral therapy for generalized anxiety disorder: a preliminary randomized controlled trial. *Journal of Anxiety Disorders.* 2009;23:1106–1117.

28. Buckner JD, Schmidt NB. A randomized pilot study of motivation enhancement therapy to increase utilization of cognitive-behavior therapy for social anxiety. *Behaviour Research and Therapy.* 2009;47:710–715.

29. Marker I, Norton PJ. The efficacy of incorporating motivational interviewing to cognitive behavioral therapy for anxiety disorders: a review and meta-analysis. *Clin Psychology Rev.* 2018;62:1–10.

30. Dillard PK, Zuniga JA, Holstad MM. An integrative review of the efficacy of motivational interviewing in HIV management. *Patient Educ Couns.* 2017;100:636–646.

31. Chen X, Murphy DA, Naa-King S, Parsons JT. A clinic-based motivational intervention improves condom use among subgroups of youth living with HIV. *Journal of Adolescent Health*. 2011;49:193–198.

32. Holstad MM, DiIorio C, Kelley ME, Resnicow K, Sharma S. Group motivational interviewing to promote adherence to antiretroviral medications and risk reduction behaviors in HIV infected women. *AIDS Behav*. 2011;15:885–896.

33. Naar-King S, Parsons JT, Murphy D, Kolmodin K, Harris DR. A multisite randomized trial of a motivational intervention targeting multiple risks in youth living with HIV: initial effects on motivation, self-efficacy, and depression. *Journal of Adolescent Health*. 2010;46:422–428.

34. Schaefer MR, Kavookjian J. The impact of motivational interviewing on adherence and symptom severity in adolescents and young adults with chronic illness: a systematic review. *Patient Educ Couns*. 2018;100:2190–2199.

35. Lovejoy TI. Telephone-delivered motivational interviewing targeting sexual risk behavior reduces depression, anxiety, and stress in HIV-positive older adults. *Ann Behav Med*. 2012;44:416–421.

SECTION IV
IMPLEMENTATION OF MOTIVATIONAL INTERVIEWING

13 Learning and Experiencing Motivational Interviewing

Jin Cheng, Claire Becker,
and Antoine Douaihy

Motivational interviewing (MI) is a conversational style that has a unique way of viewing the patient and practitioner dichotomy comparing to the traditional medical model. The role of MI in HIV care has been discussed at length in the previous chapters. The core of MI is its "spirit," which is defined by these elements: partnership, acceptance, collaboration, and evocation.[1] This is the mindset and the "heartset" underlying the practice. Understanding and experiencing the spirit of MI is the most fundamental step in the process of learning MI. Adopting the spirit of MI provides a foundation for the cumulative process of learning it.[2] The MI spirit offers a context and is well suited within the practitioner's role as a "helper." Learning how to facilitate behavior change is a rewarding and transforming experience for many practitioners: "This approach is likely to change you."[3preface] We often tend to view patients as a "set of mechanical" problems that require tuning and fixing by the practitioner; in fact, patients are individuals whose behaviors are influenced by their own value system and motivations. This can lead to high level of discord as the practitioners often attempt to impose their goals and values instead of working collaboratively with patients, focusing on patients' own goals, and respecting their autonomy. Carefully reflecting upon how we approach patients — "bedside manner" — is an essential component in evaluating practitioner's knowledge, skills and attitudes toward MI.

CHALLENGES OF LEARNING MOTIVATIONAL INTERVIEWING

MI is a skill set in the locked clinical tool box that needs the "heartset" to unlock its full potential. One of the most challenging, yet rewarding, aspects of learning MI is to ensure that practitioners receive regular supervision and coaching. So crucial to have mentorship while learning MI, particularly since so much of learning MI is experiential. Furthermore, a proper mentorship fit provides pause to the hurried accumulation of skills that derails so many practitioners.[2] It is not unusual to quickly move to the next set of skills—as is common in learning most medical procedural skills acquisition—without going through guided self-reflection on that particular skill to assure that it was learned and practiced thoroughly. A mentor is extremely helpful in addressing challenging situations and providing guidance during the process of learning. No matter what metric or evaluation tool is used, there are subtleties of language and behavior for any practitioner that can only be addressed through observation and in vivo coaching by a skilled supervisor.

Learning MI is also a collaborative process that is enriched by shared learning. As practitioners progress through the learning process, it is important to share these experiences and with your colleagues and trainees. Collaboration with colleagues invites candid sharing with the end goal of expanding the practice repertoire and strengthening self-efficacy in the process of counseling patients on behavior change. This is exemplified in role-plays and practice group exercises that allow practitioners to assume the role of the patient, practitioner, and feedback provider.

STAGES IN LEARNING MOTIVATIONAL INTERVIEWING

First introduced by Miller and Moyers[4] in a seminal paper in 2006, the underlying concept was to create a helpful framework to customize training for practitioners by using 8 stages that progress through to establish competence in the practice of MI. The stages are points in training where practitioners may struggle and get stuck. These stages tend to overlap. Identifying the stage of learning and attending to its challenges can be useful in facilitating continued advancement as practitioners go through training in MI.

Stage 1: The Spirit of Motivational Interviewing

Practitioners get stuck when they are not open to the spirit of MI and have assumptions about patients or about their role in clinical encounters. This can lead to discord in the encounter resulting in the practitioner becoming confrontational, overly directive, or overly advising. The early-stage practitioner must understand the importance of being open to the spirit and how the spirit defines and guides the MI approach.

Stage 2: OARS Skills

The skills that are required for doing competent motivational interviewing session can be summarized as open-ended questions, affirmations, reflections and summarizations (OARS). Reflective listening is a challenging skill to master and being able to consistently engage in requires continuous development. Practitioners are mostly used to asking questions to gather data and struggle to recognize the therapeutic impact of reflective listening.

Stage 3: Recognizing Change Talk

This stage is distinctive to MI. Paying attention to patient's change talk is crucial in mobilizing behavior change. Practitioners are charged with helping the patient to resolve ambivalence and elicit motivations for change. It is important to key in to change talk—desire, ability, need, and reasons (DARN) and commitment, activation, and taking steps (CAT statements)—that favors movement toward change.

Stage 4: Eliciting and Strengthening Change Talk

The ability to actively elicit and reinforce change talk distinguishes MI from other counseling modalities. Recognizing and facilitating change talk occurs through repeated reflections, affirmations, and open-ended questions, thereby continuously evoking reasons for change. Change talk must be supported by a clear intent and gentle guidance from the trainee. Frequent change talk expressed by the patient shows the practitioner is on the right track and is an accessible feedback mechanism for the practitioner to guide the session.

Stage 5: Responding to Sustain Talk: Rolling with Resistance

This is different from confronting or opposing sustain talk (as the status quo). The proper approach is to not elicit sustain talk but neither to ignore it. Rather allow and accept it. If you attempt to negate sustain talk by directly challenging it, it will come back stronger. You can reflect it, and often you will get change talk as a result. Supporting patient's autonomy leads to less discord in the encounter.

Stage 6: Developing a Change Plan

Transitioning from change talk to planning for change requires tact and timing. As the patient's expresses more significant, it could indicate a good timing toward developing a plan of action. In fact, patients will be your best teacher on when the timing is appropriate. If patient still expresses some ambivalence, exploring deeper would be helpful before proceeding to the change plan conversation. This process should feel more like dancing than wrestling. This can be described as collaborative brainstorming while being in the patient's shoes.

Stage 7: Consolidating Commitment

Once the practitioner and the patient developed a change plan, the practitioner's approach would be to focus on strengthening patient's commitment. It is important that the patient become responsible for this specific commitment to change. Emphasizing autonomy remains crucial.

Stage 8: Integration of MI with Other Modalities

MI was never intended as a be-all, end-all therapeutic method, or even as a long-term therapy. Yet, MI must be used first, and throughout treatment, because of its importance as a style for relating to patients. The MI style assumes nothing about the symptom, problem or issue at hand. Rather, MI leaves it to the patient to define it. As this is accomplished and ambivalence is reduced, behavior change treatment works optimally when MI is integrated with other therapeutic modalities. Together, for example, cognitive-behavioral therapy (CBT) and MI change plans because CBT provides the technology for how change is implemented.

TRAINING COMPONENTS IN MOTIVATIONAL INTERVIEWING

The necessary ingredients for high-quality training include instruction, practice, feedback, and in vivo coaching, and modeling. We will elaborate on all these components and incorporate experiences shared by practitioners.

Why Train in MI?

1. It is an evidence-based approach and focuses on a patient's motivation, commitment, and planning for behavioral change, and it works for a wide variety of behaviors, particularly in the context of HIV care such as adherence to antiretroviral regimens, engagement in treatment, substance use, and other medical issues experienced by PLWH.
2. MI is simple enough so that practitioners can gain competence in using it with 4 weeks of intensive training.
3. MI is complicated enough that one can put in a lifetime of work perfecting the use of the approach.
4. Patients feel respected, heard, and more willing to make lifelong changes.
5. Brief motivational interventions can have a major impact on behavior change.
6. MI can be used as a clinical style, a freestanding therapeutic approach, and/or integrated with any other treatment modalities as we have discussed in the context of HIV care in other sections of the book.

It is important for beginning practitioners to learn one therapeutic approach well to start off. Practitioners who can learn to competently provide one approach to working with patients can begin to see their interventions as either adherent or nonadherent to the therapeutic model. When practitioners notice they have deviated from the therapeutic frame of the model, they can figure out why they did it and whether it was helpful or unhelpful (e.g., if they are providing nondirective approach and they become highly directive). The adherence to therapeutic modalities (i.e., fidelity) also informs the practitioners know when the patient deviates from the therapeutic frame and cues them to investigate these deviations.

First, *instruction* is fluid. It involves book learning and watching videos. Many resources are available at www.motivationalinterviewing.org. In a learning clinical interdisciplinary environment, practitioners listen, read, and get an intellectual sense of what MI is about. In these settings, practitioners can also teach each other about basic elements of MI. Instruction and knowledge alone are not enough and do not change practice. People may think they learn to deliver counseling from instruction, but they don't.

Practice involves the use and repetition of skill. One way of practicing is through training workshops that are available at various skill levels in most of the United States and other countries. Such workshops provide opportunity to practice skills and learn from engaging in role-plays and real plays. Practitioners may practice different skills without greatly improving them. They can practice mindlessly or mindfully. Deliberate practice feels effortful. It requires focus and attunement to rough areas and striving toward improvement. Deliberate practice is practicing something that is beyond people's current ability. Repetition is focused on breaking down skills (i.e., reflective listening, evocative questions) into basic units and improving on each of those chunks and then continually practicing these skills at more challenging levels. Interestingly, it takes about 10,000 hours of deliberate practice to become an expert at anything. Research found that deliberate practice predicts performance well above anything that we would call innate or genetic talent.[5] A typical research study on deliberate practice in music finds that when we divide musicians into the top third and bottom third of skill level, as rated by their teachers, what divides them more than anything is the amount and quality of daily practice.[6] The goal of training is not to make practitioners "experts" in MI, but why not structure the practice of MI and other therapeutic skills to be deliberate practice, rather than just repetition. If we practice MI but we fail to do the deliberate practice, that could create a challenge in making progress in strengthening skills. "Practice in practice" means practitioners take their learning, and their feedback, and practice once in clinical settings with others observing and listening. This could enhance the learning collaborative experience. From our clinical experiences providing training and supervision, practitioners have repeatedly expressed fulfillment and increased self-efficacy and showed major improvements in their skills that they attributed to intensive deliberate practice.

- "Real learning occurs when you extend past your limit and make mistakes, right?"
- "The biggest effect was that it really made me want to up my game. I think having people observing me doing the session caused me to develop more internal awareness of everything I was saying/doing and how it was impacting my patient. It was initially tough to have that going on while also trying to do counseling. Over time, that process became more automatic, and I think it's that process that really helps me to be able to continue to use MI now that I'm not getting feedback every day."

Most practitioners tend to be inaccurate at assessing their own performance. They tend to think they're doing better than they are. In a way, living without feedback helps people keep this problematic thinking. *Feedback* and in vivo *coaching* are an assessment of practitioners' work with a focus on how they can improve it and where their challenges are. Feedback provides practitioners with a map for their deliberate practice. Miller and Rollnick[1] found that with modest amount of expert coaching, practitioners can improve their MI proficiency. MI coaching need to be based on direct observation such as in-person coaching and/or reviewing media recordings. In a group setting, this can be an effective way of experiencing MI as practitioners get feedback on their encounters with patients and at the same time they can provide feedback for other team members. The best feedback, as reported by practitioners, provides examples of what to work on, how to work on it, and how it might look when it is finished. Feedback has been shown to be vital for MI training. There is strong research evidence showing that instruction with feedback, coaching, or both raises practitioners' performance to competence in MI, whereas instruction alone tends not to raise performance.[7] Individuals who had only completed the instructional part thought they improved a great deal, and in fact they were less likely to want to engage in more training because they felt they had already learned MI, even though they really had not. This is an important caution—if practitioners don't put themselves out there for feedback, they can think they have something mastered that they are actually incompetent in doing! Developing elite performance related to feedback and deliberate practice is known as a growth mindset, a construct developed by Dweck.[8] Real and honest feedback, as well as other elements of training, fosters a growth mindset. In our practice, the feedback the practitioners receive from us and their peers is consistently delivered in an approach, using the MI spirit with specifics about MI adherent and nonadherent practices and how/what can be improved.

"If we create a culture of showing our work and soliciting constructive feedback, we are acknowledging that looking at our flaws and errors is important to getting better. This is how we do a better job, and this is how we can do better for our clients." This is a perspective expressed by a clinical psychology intern.

The benefits of a growth mindset include the following.[8]

- Challenge is fun rather than terrifying (if you must show yourself and everyone your intelligence, challenges are a threat).
- People with a growth mindset tend to be better at identifying their strengths and weaknesses, whereas those with a fixed mindset tend to overestimate their abilities.
- You can, and must, make mistakes rather than needing to be perfect.
- People with a growth mindset feel smart when faced with challenge, while those with a fixed mindset feel stressed and stupid.
- Those with a fixed mindset tend to have a more fragile self-esteem and are at higher risk for depression.
- Randomly assigning people to a fixed or growth mindset condition in a computer training course, researchers found that those with fixed mindset lost confidence in their computer skills, while those in the growth mindset condition gained confidence.

I quickly became accustomed to receiving feedback and in vivo coaching as well as offering it, though both were uncomfortable at first. Through this constructive team environment, we pushed each other to excel, take risks, and be honest about our perceived struggles/successes. It was so much fun to watch each other's MI skills progress.

The development of the growth mindset is exactly what the practitioner in the previous example describes. She says that at first it was hard to accept this feedback and difficult to be accustomed to that, but that, with time, it became more comfortable. This use of struggles/successes is a perfect description of the growth mindset—"if you struggle, you succeed."

The feedback during my six weeks of immersing myself in clinical training on an addiction unit was an essential part of learning MI and embracing its spirit. We had a supportive and keen team and pushed each other to work hard and do our best every day. . . . Coaching helped me grasp how to mobilize the process of change once the patient is expressing change talk and commitment language. An incredibly effective strategy was to "go deeper" with my reflections (e.g., to take more risks with my hypotheses of the underlying meaning of a patient's words). This set the stage for using more powerful, evocative questions, and many of my patients really embraced exploring their internal worlds and external interactions.

Something that we find incredibly helpful in training in MI is *modeling*. Put simply, modeling shows what therapeutic work can look like. It takes a while to begin to approximate that model. Practitioners are encouraged to learn MI through modeling without losing the identity of their clinical style.

Watching my mentor's sessions was a fundamental part of how I learned MI. I felt like I was in a concert hall, watching a conductor fervently evoke music from the orchestra. . . . I also took in a lot through observation of body language and tone. In many sessions, I would write down what I felt were particularly effective/ evocative phrasings and review them later. I think one of the benefits of having an MI mentor is that like any apprenticeship, you observe their skills and techniques and incorporate/deliver these through your own personal style.

As articulated by one of our medical trainees:

We need to develop an atmosphere of continual improvement—where we are going with best practices rather than status quo. We're trying solutions that are on the cutting edge of research. I think the most important things we should challenge ourselves to do are to truly challenge ourselves and those around us to have the utmost respect for our patients, to drop judgments and build our accurate empathy skills, and to truly listen and understand where someone is and allow ourselves to be hopeful of where they can go. MI is particularly well suited as a framework for this type of work.

EVIDENCE-BASED TOOLS FOR PROVIDING FEEDBACK

Feedback and coaching in MI should focus on training practitioners in skills that can be reliably measured. This resulted in the development of several tools routinely used in the evaluation and feedback of trainees. Common to all these tools is attention to the spirit of MI and a focus on a particular target behavior in the clinical interaction. It is beyond the scope of this chapter to provide extensive details of these tools. Please see the references for more details. The following is a brief overview of the most practical tools:

Motivational Interviewing Treatment Integrity Scale

This a coding system that focus on the practitioner's specific MI skills and spirit. The most recent version of this scale is Motivational Interviewing Treatment Integrity Scale (MITI) 4.2.1 (9). The MITI has 2 components: the global scores and the behavior counts. The grading is based on global ratings on cultivating change talk, softening sustain talk, partnership, and empathy on a scale of 1 to 5, where 1 is the lowest and 5 is the highest. The second component captures specific practitioner behavior counts of MI and non-MI adherent behaviors without regard to how they fit into the overall impression of the practitioner's use of MI: giving information, persuade or persuade with permission, question, reflection simple or complex reflection, affirm, seeking collaboration, emphasizing autonomy, and confront. The initial intent was to provide a measure of treatment integrity for clinical trials of MI and a means of providing formal, structured feedback. It is the most commonly used tool for assessing MI adherence of a counseling session and for providing feedback for the practitioner.

Behavioral Change Counseling Index

Behavior change counseling (BCC)[10] is an adaptation of MI that is a brief intervention primarily used in healthcare settings. It is designed to help patients discuss the how and why of change and help them understand how their perceptions of current situations affect their behaviors and choices for behavior change. The difference between BCC and MI is that MI is focused on eliciting change talk and developing discrepancy while BCC is focused on simply listening and understanding the patient's perspective to determine how best to guide the patient to behavior change. From this adaptation, the Behavioral Change Counseling Index (BECCI) was developed as a 12-item scale that measures specific MI behaviors for the provision of feedback in both practical and research settings. It is the first instrument specifically developed to assess health behavior change, while incorporating measures of skills used in both MI and BCC. The focus of the BECCI is on trainee's consulting behavior and attitude and not the behaviors of the patient. It is designed to be scored easily and quickly, given the time constraints of the healthcare setting.

Helpful Responses Questionnaire

The Helpful Responses Questionnaire (HRQ)[11] is one of the older and more frequently used scales when evaluating MI skills and behavior. It was developed to assess the use of empathic language. HRQ is a brief, free-response questionnaire that can be administered to groups or individuals. It consists of 6 scenarios of simulated patient interactions that are likely to be seen in clinical settings. After each scenario, the practitioner is instructed to play the role of the counselor and provide a helpful response. The average administration time is approximately 15 to 20 minutes.

REFERENCES

1. Miller WR, Rollnick S. *Motivational interviewing: Helping people change.* 3rd ed. New York, NY: Guilford Press; 2013.
2. Douaihy A, Kelly TM, Gold, MA. *Motivational Interviewing: A guide for medical trainees.* New York, NY: Oxford University Press; 2014.
3. Miller WR, Rollnick S. *Motivational Interviewing: Preparing People to* Change Addictive. New York, NY: Guilford Press; 1991.
4. Miller WR, Moyers TB. Eight stages in learning motivational interviewing. *J Teaching Addictions.* 2006;5(1):3–17.
5. Macnamara BN, Hambrick DZ, Oswald FL. Deliberate practice and performance in music, games, sports, education, and professions: a meta-analysis. *Psychol. Sci.* 2014;25(8):1608–1618.
6. Platz F, Kopiez R, Lehmann AC, Wolf A. The influence of deliberate practice on musical achievement: a meta-analysis. *Front Psychol.* 2014;5:646.
7. Schwalbe CS, Oh HY, Zweben A. Sustaining motivational interviewing; a meta-analysis of training studies. *Addiction.* 2014;109(8):1287–1294.

8. Dweck C. *Mindset: How You Can Fulfill Your Potential*. London, England: Constable and Robinson; 2012.

9. Moyers TB, Manuel JK, Ernest D. Motivational interviewing treatment integrity coding manual 4.1. Unpublished manual. 2014.

10. Lane C, Huws-Thomas M, Hood K, et al. Measuring adaptations of motivational interviewing: the development and validation of the behaviour change counselling index (BECCI). *Patient Educ Couns*. 2005;56:166–173.

11. Miller WR, Hendrick KE, Orlofsky DR. The Helpful Responses Questionnaire: A procedure for measuring therapeutic empathy. *J Clin Psychol*. 1991;47(3):444–448.

14 Motivational Interviewing in Global Practice Settings

The Importance of Ongoing Support

Sarah Dewing and Cathy Mathews

BACKGROUND

Motivational interviewing (MI) has demonstrated efficacy in promoting positive behavior change and is widely promoted for use in healthcare settings. There is evidence that brief training leads to an improvement in healthcare providers' MI skills[1,2] but to what extent does MI training then impact healthcare practitioners every day practice? The implementation of evidence-based practice is a well-known challenge, and health research findings often fail to translate in to practice and in to meaningful patient outcomes.[3] The barriers to the implementation of new practices and programs in healthcare settings include a focus on more urgent medical issues,[4] high workload,[5,6] a lack of time,[4,7] inadequate training,[4,6] a lack of support,[4,7] and limited resources.[8] Such barriers may be more significant in developing countries where resources for healthcare are more constrained. In this chapter, we will review and discuss the implementation and evaluation of an evidence-based MI intervention called Options for Health within a public sector, primary healthcare setting in Cape Town, South Africa. We will also focus on addressing challenges related to the transfer of newly acquired communication skills into practice as well as the importance of providing ongoing support and supervision.

OPTIONS FOR HEALTH INTERVENTION

In low- and middle-income countries, lay health workers (LHWs) are increasingly being integrated into the formal health service to expand capacity for service delivery, specifically with regard to HIV/AIDS services and support.[9,10] LHWs are individuals who have no formal professional, paraprofessional certificate or degreed tertiary education, but who carry out functions related to healthcare delivery.[11] At the time of our study, one of the main strategies for supporting antiretroviral therapy adherence was individual counseling delivered by LHWs working within public health clinics.

To strengthen the standard-of-care counseling program, we trained lay counselors in Options, a brief counseling intervention based on MI. The project was referred to as Options for Health: Western Cape (Options: WC), and the Options model was intended to replace the adherence counseling model that was being practiced at the time. The model being implemented before Options was in theory client-centered and focused on problem management, but research showed that the relationship between counselors and patients was characterized by high provider control and authority and that counseling sessions tended to take the form of information-based health education.[12-14] Further, counselors contravened core principles of client-centered counseling by issuing warnings, being confrontational, moralizing, casting judgements and patronizing patients.[15]

Options for Health consists of 8 steps in which the counselor (i) introduces the discussion, (ii) assesses the client's risk behavior, (iii) assesses importance and confidence to evaluate the client's readiness to change their behavior, (iv) decides whether to focus on importance or confidence, (v) identifies barriers to behavior change and works to elicit change talk, (vi) discusses strategies for change, (vii) negotiates an action plan, and (viii) documents the session for follow-up.[16] We trained 39 lay ART adherence counselors from 21 clinics around Cape Town to implement the intervention with their nonadherent patients. Of counselors taking part in our study, only 26 had completed grade 12 schooling and spoke either Xhosa ($n = 27$) or Afrikaans ($n = 8$) as a first language.

TRANSLATING RESEARCH TO PRACTICE

In moving an intervention from research into practice settings, it is recommended that training approximate naturalistic training conditions and is typical of the training provided under ordinary circumstances.[17] As such, Options training was conducted in English; Xhosa and Afrikaans translations for key concepts were generated in collaboration by facilitators and participants. Counselors were divided into 2 groups and trained over 2 consecutive weeks (5 days; 35 hours for each group). The first day of training focused on the communication skills and principles associated with MI, including ambivalence, readiness to change, change talk and resistance, reflective listening, asking permission before giving information or advice, open- and closed-ended questions, and providing information in a manner consistent with MI (elicit–provide–elicit).[15] The MI module was delivered by 2 local experts in MI with experience in training lay counselors in the approach, one of whom was also fluent in Xhosa. The remaining 4 days of training focused on learning the steps of the Options protocol with continued emphasis on the use of MI-consistent micro skills and techniques. Teaching methods used included didactic presentations and handouts, experiential learning exercises, modeling (by facilitators and in video demonstrations) and role-play.

Following initial training, we collected audio-recordings of counseling sessions conducted with clinic patients for transcription, translation in to English and analysis.[15] Counselors' adherence to the Options protocol was evaluated using a coding sheet developed by us, while their proficiency in MI was measured using the Motivational Interviewing Treatment Integrity (MITI) tool, Version 3.0. This instrument is appropriate for assessing entry-level competence in MI.[18] In terms of fidelity to the Options protocol, only 23% of counselors conducted steps 1 through 7 (the completion of step

8 was not assessed). Also, some steps that were completed were not always completed well: counselors struggled with those steps representing the more strategic elements of MI, namely, assessing readiness to change, choosing the appropriate construct to focus on, and facilitating change talk (Options steps 3 to 5). Despite struggling with some of the 7 steps, 80% of counselors facilitated a discussion with the client around strategies for behavior change. As a group, counselors failed to meet the suggested thresholds for beginning proficiency in MI as measured by the MITI 3.0.[18] They displayed particularly low levels of empathy and did not approach the client as the active decision maker in the interaction. Counselors were successful in maintaining an appropriate focus on a specific target behavior (referred to as "direction" in the MITI 3.0). Importantly, high scores on direction do not necessarily indicate a better use of MI[18] and, in this case, were likely a result of the high level of provider control that characterized interactions prior to the Options: WC program. In terms of micro-counseling skills as measured by the MITI 3.0, counselors relied heavily on closed-ended questions, simple reflections, and the provision of information. Most counselors made statements that were deemed to be inconsistent with the spirit and approach of MI (these include advising without permission, confronting and giving orders, commands or imperatives).

Refresher training and supervision focused on upskilling are not provided to lay counselors as a part of the standard-of-care lay counseling program. Because Options: WC had been intended to be implemented in the way it would be rolled out if the local public health authorities were to implement it, ongoing technical support was not included in our original implementation plan. During implementation it became clear that additional support was necessary, and so we delivered a 2-day (14 hour) refresher training course at 4 months following the initial training. At 5 months following the refresher training, we implemented monthly Options-specific supervision sessions over a 4-month period.[15] Supervision was delivered in a small-group format for 1 hour. Each month sessions focused on recapping the Options protocol, MI principles, communication skills, and techniques. Twelve months following the initial Options training course (referred to as Time 2), we again collected audio recordings of counseling sessions for transcription, translation, and analysis. In total, we were able to compare performance after the initial training (Time 1) to performance at Time 2 for 22 counselors.[15] We saw that counselors' performance was improved about some aspects of Options, but not others. Counselors continued to experience difficulty with those parts of the protocol requiring a conceptual understanding of MI principles, that is, steps 3 to 5. In contrast to the low impact of refresher training and supervision on the more strategic elements of MI and the Options 8-step protocol is the impact it had on counselors' proficiency in the more basic elements of MI. Counselors' practice at Time 2 was significantly more like MI in terms of the spirit with which counseling was delivered. Our data showed a significant difference in the extent to which counselors approached their patients as equal partners in the interaction and with an understanding that motivation (and the ability) for change lie within the client. Counselors were observed to be significantly more empathetic and improved in their use of micro-counseling skills such as open-ended questions and reflections. Further, we observed a substantial increase in the number of individual counselors achieving not only beginning proficiency but also competency in MI adherent behavior (from 18% [$n = 4$] at Time 1 to 50% [$n = 11$] at Time 2) and a decrease in MI nonadherent behavior. MI adherent behaviors include asking permission before giving information or advice, affirming the clients' self-efficacy, emphasizing the clients control and offering supportive statements.[18] This improvement is meaningful because the avoidance of MI inconsistent behavior may be of primary importance in effecting positive patient outcomes.[19,20] Another positive finding is that counselors maintained a focus on problem-solving in their counseling sessions.

Evidence-based strategies such as MI have the potential to improve the delivery of health services, but the failure of providers to develop sufficient competence in the approach may be a significant barrier to the transfer of MI into practice. Our research shows that lay counselors were able to conduct counseling in accordance with the central tenets of the MI approach, but that ongoing technical support was necessary for them to achieve skill proficiency and to support skills transfer. Skills transfer is an ongoing and dynamic process,[21] and it is likely difficult to suppress prior counseling habits and practices that may be inconsistent with MI.[22] Indeed, research published in the years since the Options: WC project indicates that MI skills learned in training deteriorate over time if posttraining support is not provided.[2] This is true for a range of healthcare providers, including medical professionals. The requirements for effective ongoing support appear to be modest: while our research did not allow us to separate out the effects of refresher training from those of monthly supervision, a recent meta-analysis of MI training studies found that as little as 5 hours of contact over a 6-month period was sufficient to sustain MI skills learnt in training. Of course, different types of healthcare provider may benefit more or less from different delivery methods. For example, in their study investigating the relationship between healthcare provider characteristics and the acquisition of MI skills, Carpenter and colleagues[23] found that providers with a university degree benefited most from supervision based on coaching around audio-recorded counseling sessions, while trainees without a degree benefited most from coaching combined with more immediate in vivo supervision.

CONCLUSIONS

Much work has been put into developing and testing the efficacy of theory-based prevention interventions, including those based on MI strategies. While it is generally recognized that the efficacy of a program does not guarantee its effectiveness in practice, there is still an assumption that evidence-based interventions can be easily transferred into real-world settings.[24] The Options: WC project is an example of just how difficult it can be to move a program from research in to practice. One of the main lessons we learned was the importance of ongoing supervision for ensuring provider competency and encouraging the transfer of learned skills into practice. As an advanced counseling technique, the introduction of MI into a new practice setting is likely to represent a change in practice from standard-of-care communication and counseling strategies. Ongoing technical support needs to be included as an integral part of any implementation program.

REFERENCES

1. Barwick MA, Bennett LM, Johnson SN, McGowan J, Moore, JE. Training health and mental health professionals in motivational interviewing: A systematic review. *Child Youth Serv Rev.* 2012;34(9):1786–1795.

2. Schwalbe CS, Oh HY, Zweben A. Sustaining motivational interviewing: a meta-analysis of training studies. *Addiction.* 2014;109(8):1287–1294.

3. Damschroder LJ, Aron DC, Keith RE, Kirsh SR, Alexander JA, Lowery JC. Fostering implementation of health services research findings into practice: a consolidated framework for advancing implementation science. *Implement Sci.* 2009;4:50.

4. Whitlock EP, Orleans CT, Pender N, Allan J. Evaluating primary care behavioral counseling interventions: an evidence-based approach. *Am J Prev Med.* 2002;22(4):267–284.

5. Grol R, Grimshaw J. From best evidence to best practice: effective implementation of change in patients' care. *Lancet.* 2003;362(9391):1225–1230.

6. Johnson M, Jackson R, Guillaume L, Meier P, Goyder E. Barriers and facilitators to implementing screening and brief intervention for alcohol misuse: a systematic review of qualitative evidence. *J Public Health.* 2011;33(3):412–421.

7. Franks H, Hardiker NR, Mcgrath M, Mcquarrie C. Public health interventions and behaviour change: reviewing the grey literature. *Public Health.* 2012;126(1):12–17.

8. Dane AV, Schneider BH. Program integrity in primary and early secondary prevention: Are implementation effects out of control? *Clin Psych Rev.* 1998;18(1):23–45.

9. Schneider H, Hlophe H, van Rensburg D. Community health workers and the response to HIV/AIDS in South Africa: tensions and prospects. *Health Policy Plan.* 2008;23(3):179–187.

10. Thurling CH, Harris C. Prevention of mother to child transmission lay counsellors: Are they adequately trained?. *Curationis.* 2012;35(1):64.

11. Lewin SA, Dick J, Pond P, et al. Lay health workers in primary and community health care. *Cochrane Database Syst Rev.* 2005;(1):CD004015.

12. Buskens I, Jaffe A. Demotivating infant feeding counselling encounters in Southern Africa: Do counsellors need more or different training? *AIDS Care.* 2008;20(3):337–345.

13. Dewing S, Mathews C, Schaay N, Cloete A, Louw, J, Simbayi L. "It's important to take your medication everyday okay?" An evaluation of counselling by lay counsellors for ARV adherence support in the Western Cape, South Africa. *AIDS Behav.* 2013;*17*(1):203–212.

14. Richter L, Durrheim K, Griesel D, Solomon V, van Rooyen H. Evaluation of HIV/AIDS counselling in South Africa. Contract report submitted to the Department of Health. Pietermaritzburg, South Africa: School of Psychology, University of Natal; 1999.

15. Dewing S, Mathews C, Cloete A, et al. From research to practice: lay adherence counsellors' fidelity to an evidence-based intervention for promoting adherence to antiretroviral treatment in the Western cape, South Africa. *AIDS Behav.* 2013;17(9):2935–2945.

16. Cornman DH, Christie S, Amico KR, Cruess S, Shepherd, L. *Options Intervention Protocol Manual: A Step-by-Step Guide to Risk Reduction Counselling with PLWHA.* Storss, CT: University of Connecticut; 2007.

17. Roy-Byrne PP, Sherbourne CD, Craske MG, et al. Moving treatment research from clinical trials to the real world. *Psychiatr Serv.* 2003;54(3):327–332.

18. Moyers TB, Martin T, Manuel JK, Miller RW, Ernst D. Revised global scales: Motivational Interviewing Treatment Integrity 3.0 (MITI 3.0). Center on Alcoholism, Substance Abuse and Addictions. https://casaa.unm.edu/download/miti3_1.pdf. Revised January 22, 2010.

19. Apodaca TR, Longabaugh R. Mechanisms of change in motivational interviewing: A review and preliminary evaluation of the evidence. *Addiction.* 2009;104(5):705–715.

20. Gaume J, Gmel G, Faouzi M, Daeppen JB. Counselor skill influences outcomes of brief motivational interventions. *J Subst Abuse Treat.* 2009;37(2):151–159.

21. Van den Eertwegh V, Van Dulmen S, Van Dalen J, Scherpbier AJ, Van der Vleuten CP. Learning in context: identifying gaps in research on the transfer of medical communication skills to the clinical workplace. *Patient Educ Couns.* 2013;90(2):184–192.

22. Söderlund LL, Nilsen P, Kristensson M. Learning motivational interviewing: Exploring primary health care nurses" training and counselling experiences. *Health Educ J.* 2008;67(2):102–109.
23. Carpenter KM, Cheng WY, Smith JL, et al. "Old dogs" and new skills: how clinician characteristics relate to motivational interviewing skills before, during, and after training. *J Consult Clin Psychol.* 2012;80(4):560–573.
24. Hirschhorn LR, Ojikutu B, Rodriguez W. Research for change: using implementation research to strengthen HIV care and treatment scale-up in resource-limited settings. *J Infect Dis.* 2007;196(Suppl 3):S516–S522.

15 Integration of Motivational Interviewing with Other Intervention Modalities in HIV Care

Marcia M. Holstad

BACKGROUND

Because HIV is now a chronic treatable condition, self-management behaviors are increasingly important for patients to maintain a long healthy life. MI can be used by providers to discuss behavior change and tailor self-management behaviors with the ultimate goal of improving and maintaining quality of life. Often MI has been integrated with other treatment modalities such as providing individualized feedback on questionnaires or diaries, cognitive-behavioral therapy (CBT) within a group setting, and health education. An innovative use combines MI with emerging technologies. Probably the most frequently cited self-management behaviors addressed in research using MI in people living with HIV (PLWH) have been antiretroviral therapy (ART) medication adherence and safer sex; however, MI has been effective for reduction of substance use, cigarette smoking, alcohol use, depression, and anxiety in this population.

Interventions that combine MI with other modalities seem to have somewhat stronger findings. One MI-based intervention combined 2 face-to-face sessions delivered by trained health educators with an educational audiotape and booklet provided before the session and a letter sent 2 weeks afterward that summarized the participants' goals and adherence self-management strategies. Adherence improved in intervention participants and decreased in the health education control group after 3 months follow-up, however results did not reach statistical significance. Although more intervention participants achieved undetectable viral loads (52% vs. 44%), the results were not statistically significant but were nonetheless clinically meaningful. The MI participants also reported more self-management behaviors and had improved attitudes about their ART.[1] This study was conducted within a clinic setting and could be adapted by practitioners or clinic health educators. Health education materials are readily available and in combination with MI could boost patient understanding of the importance and effectiveness of ART and implementation of personal self-management strategies such as setting goals for medication-taking, devising tailored reminder strategies, and adherence to appointments.

Parsons and colleagues[2] conducted eight 60-minute sessions of individually delivered MI plus cognitive behavioral skills intervention with hazardous drinkers with HIV. The sessions focused on both medication adherence and reduction of drinking and were tailored to the participant's behaviors. Sessions included education, self-assessment, skill building, practice, and take-home activities. Compared to health education, they demonstrated improved adherence and clinical outcomes of CD4 count and viral load at 3 months; however, the effect was not sustained at six months follow-up. All participants decreased drinking over the 6-month period.

Goggin and colleagues[3] tested MI in combination with CBT (MI + CBT) and MI plus CBT plus modified directly observed therapy (MI + CBT + mDOT) and found an improvement in adherence in the MI + CBT + mDOT group at 12 weeks, which steeply declined as mDOT was tapered and withdrawn. Although implementation of observed therapy may be cost- and time-prohibitive for most clinics, patients at high risk could be considered for such a program, acknowledging that when the administration ceases, adherence might also decline. The authors report a dose effect in that nonadherence decreased as the number of sessions of MI + CBT or MI + CBT + mDOT attended increased. Addition of booster MI sessions that focus on personal adherence strategies after removal of mDOT could increase adherence. One clinic in a large southern city that serves high-risk, vulnerable patients with HIV illness employs a similar type of intervention in an in-clinic transition center for patients with HIV and severe mental illness. Patients can store their meds at the center and return daily for medication administration, social support, therapeutic counseling, and other services provided by psychologists, social workers, and nurses. In this center, MI is integrated into the therapeutic milieu.

In an innovative project, MI was incorporated into a music-based messaging program, the LIVE Network.[4] In this simulated and recorded disc jockey talk show, the disc jockey posed questions from callers to HIV providers who used MI in their responses. Over the course of the program, the disc jockey interspersed 10 songs, written and produced to educate and motivate patients to deal with issues that impact medication adherence and symptom management. In this pilot project, compared to usual care controls, participants who received the LIVE Network program had higher adherence (pill counts, plasma antiretroviral drug levels in therapeutic range). LIVE Network participants also had reductions in viral load and increased self-efficacy over 12 weeks of follow-up.

MI, either alone or in combination with other strategies (CBT, health education), has been very effective in promoting safer sex and reduction in sexual risk behaviors in several studies and populations including HIV-positive men and women,[5] older adults,[6] youth and young adults,[7-9] and persons in South Africa.[10]

SafeTalk[1,5] was a multicomponent, individually administered intervention designed to reduce risky sexual behaviors. It included 4 MI sessions in tandem with an educational CD and booklet that participants reviewed prior to the session. Booster letters that summarized sessions were also sent to participants after each session. There was a significantly reduced number of unprotected sex acts with at-risk partners at 8- and 12-month follow-ups, while the controls (heart healthy education) increased the number of unprotected sex acts. The SafeTalk investigators also reported a dose effect: as the number of sessions attended increased, there was an increase in self-efficacy for safer sex and reduction of unprotected anal or vaginal sex.[11,12]

Healthy Choices was a 4-session, individually administered MI intervention with individual feedback on baseline responses for 2 of 3 risk behaviors (poor adherence, substance use, sexual risk) in HIV-positive youth aged 16 to 24.[9] It was delivered over a 10-week period. After 3-months follow-up there were no differences between the control and MI participants in alcohol or marijuana use, but depression scores were significantly improved in the MI participants. Those who received at least 2 of the 4 sessions significantly improved their motivational readiness to change.[9] After 6 months, viral loads were improved for the intervention group, but this was not sustained.[8] At 15 months follow-up, those youth in the intervention had significantly lower reported alcohol use, and they had a reduced probability of being classified as high risk for both alcohol and marijuana.[13] Healthy Choices was also effective in reducing sexual risk behaviors after 15 months follow-up. Those in the intervention had higher likelihood of being classified as persistently low sexual risk and reduced the likelihood of being categorized as delayed high sexual risk. Intervention youth categorized as persistently low sexual risk and high and growing sexual risk also had reductions in condomless sex.[7] The Healthy Choices MI intervention was also tested in Tai youth with HIV who, compared to those with general health education, had no between-group differences in sexual risk behavior, alcohol use, and condom use. The MI participants, however, showed decreases in sexual risk and increases in protected sex at 1 month, but changes weren't sustained at 6 months.[14] Young adults are the fastest-growing population of persons newly diagnosed with HIV. MI was effective in this population for important self-management behaviors, and providers who work with youth and young adults with HIV could use MI to promote adherence and reduction in risky sexual and substance use behaviors. This type of program could be integrated into existing clinics with one-to-one education or provided in a group format.

Lovejoy and colleagues[6] tested the effect of telephone delivered MI in either 4 sessions or a single session, compared to a control group (standard care), on reducing unprotected sex in HIV-positive adults age 45 and older. Those with 4 versus no or 1 session had more protected sex. In addition, both the 1- and 4-session MI calls improved depression, anxiety, and stress at 6 months compared to standard care controls.[15]

In a project funded by the National Institute of Health, a novel 4 one-to-one MI session intervention has been implemented to promote disease adjustment, coping, and advanced care planning in persons with AIDS. Sessions were conducted by specially trained nurses and provided in conjunction with early palliative care clinic appointments (Holstad, et al. Living Well Project, R01NR014054).

Group-based MI was tested by Holstad and colleagues who conducted an 8-session motivational group to promote ART adherence and risk-reduction behaviors in women with HIV in the southern United States[16] and Nigeria.[17] In the US women, the group was conducted by specially trained nurses, and participants were followed for 9 months compared to a health promotion control group. There was a dose effect such that for women who attended 7 of the 8 MI groups there was significantly higher percentage of ART doses taken on schedule at 3 months, borderline at 6 months, and not significant at the final 9-month follow-up. High-attending women also reported significantly higher use of protection during sex at 6- and 9-month follow-ups. The Nigerian groups were led by trained healthcare workers. The participants had high attendance for both the control and MI groups, and there were significantly higher self-reported adherence and use of protection during sex at the 6-month follow-up compared with the controls. We are currently providing group MI to promote adherence to a walking intervention for older PLWH with cognitive impairments (Waldrop-Valverde et al., Healing Hearts, Mending Minds in Older Persons Living with HIV, R01NR014973). Large HIV service clinics often offer multiple types of support or educational groups, and MI could be incorporated into these groups to promote self-management, healthy behaviors, or coping.

In group MI, the focus is on positive behaviors and problem-solving to develop strategies to deal with barriers to promote target behaviors. The leader guides members' interactions toward positive behavior change.[18] We have adapted OARS (open-ended questions, affirmations, reflective listening, summarizing) and other techniques such as motivation/confidence rulers, decisional balance, and values clarification to a group format. We have found that two facilitators who share leadership and troubleshoot member issues works well. A group size of 6 to 8 members is ideal to facilitate sharing and problem-solving. We use a structured outline of topics and MI group activities for each session.

MI was originally developed for use in "problem drinkers," and there is a long history of its use with these persons and substance users. Ingersoll[19] found 6 individual sessions of MI plus skill-building to be equally effective in improving ART adherence and reducing addiction severity scores as a video plus information debriefing program in a pilot study of 56 nonadherent cocaine users with HIV.[19] A project aimed at reducing drinking in PLWH compared MI and individual feedback alone, MI-feedback plus daily automated call in (HealthCall) to report drinking, and an education control condition. The greatest differences in number of drinks per day occurred in persons with alcohol dependence at 30 and 60 days in the MI plus HealthCall group. The results continued at 12 months but were not significant.[20] A pilot test of a smartphone HealthCall application plus MI showed increased participant self-monitoring engagement and similar reduced drinking after 60 days.[21]

With respect to smoking cessation, a single brief MI session, when compared to prescribed advice, showed a significant drop in mean cigarettes smoked in a day at 1 month in female smokers who are HIV positive. There was no difference between groups for the 7-day point prevalence abstinence or desire to quit, perceived difficulty, and expectation for success of quitting.[22]

Based on the previously discussed studies, MI in combination with other modalities has promise for behavior change, and these exemplars provide models for providers to implement with PLWH. For healthcare professionals who want to incorporate MI into their clinical practice with PLWH, several suggestions can be offered. MI works well when there is ambivalence for changing behavior. Thus, patients who are having difficulty with self-management behaviors related to HIV or other co-morbidities are good candidates for MI. Examples of HIV self-management behaviors include engagement and retention in HIV care, medication adherence, safer sex behaviors, reduction of alcohol and drug use, smoking cessation, diet, exercise, and mental health (depression, anxiety, and coping). MI can be an effective tool and may increase effectiveness when combined with other modalities such as CBT, standard health education, or case management. MI has been effectively administered in one-on-one sessions in person and by telephone, as well as in group sessions, although fewer studies have used this method.

An effective way to begin using MI is to incorporate the spirit of MI in *all* encounters with patients. Acknowledging the patient's autonomy at whatever stage of change they are in, attempting to see the world from their eyes, and listening in a nonjudgmental manner are key to conveying *acceptance* ("Based on your lab values, your HIV illness is not well controlled—help me understand what might be contributing to this"). Conveying that they are your priority during the short time of their visit shows *compassion* ("What, if any, concerns do you have today?"). Demonstrating you are willing to work with the patient as a partner in care to brainstorm strategies, rather than telling the patient what to do conveys spirit of *collaboration* ("What strategies have you tried to discuss condom use with your partner?"). Asking the client's perspective on motivation or confidence to change displays *evocation* ("On a scale of 0 to 10, where 0 is not at all and 10 is the highest, how confident are you that you can disclose your status to your sexual partner?"). There are some patients who may want to be told what to do and asking their opinion or permission to make suggestions may not work. When asked their opinion on what might be best for them, they may respond, "You're the doctor; you tell me." These patients are few and far between, and most patients will respond positively to being included as a partner in behavior-change strategies.

In general, 4 or more sessions of MI seem to promote better outcomes for behaviors such as safer sex, adherence, and substance use. Regular and consistent use of MI by practitioners with the same patient is optimal. For patients with chronic nonadherence or lack of behavior changes, this can be challenging since the urge to tell them what to do might be strong. Keeping an armamentarium of MI-consistent creative ways to get at reasons or problem-solve regarding solutions could alleviate this urge. Asking permission to discuss your concerns about the current behavior and providing these in nonconfrontational manner can help the patient understand consequences of the behavior. Ultimately, the patient is in control of their behavior, and recognizing their autonomy to make choices (whether positive or negative for their health) may be the appropriate response ("We've talked about the pros and cons and consequences; only you can decide what is best for you").

The following are examples of how a practitioner used MI in conversations with 2 patients. The first had been out of care, and the second includes a patient education component.

Practitioner: It looks like you've missed several clinic appointments, and it's been awhile since I've seen you. Help me understand what is keeping you from attending your appointments. (Open-ended question)

Patient: Well my car broke down, and I didn't have a way to get here.

Practitioner: You've had car trouble. What exactly happened? (Reflection followed by an open-ended question)

Patient: I needed some expensive car repairs, and I didn't have the money. There is no bus service in my county, so I didn't have the bus as a choice.

Practitioner: So, your car needed some serious and costly repairs, and you were stranded because there was no public transportation in the county you lived. (Reflection)

Patient: Yes. It was hard even getting to the grocery store.

Practitioner: You are clearly frustrated about the situation. How did you manage that? (Reflection followed by an open-ended question)

Patient: My family helped me out with rides.

Practitioner: Your family has been available for you. Had you thought about contacting friends or family for a ride to clinic? (Reflection followed by a closed question)

Patient: They don't know my diagnosis and with this being a clinic for people with HIV, I didn't want to ask anyone to drive me.

Practitioner: So, you didn't want to be in a situation where disclosure of your status could occur. What other options have you considered? (Reflection followed by an open-ended question)

Patient: None that I can think of. I can't afford a taxi.

Practitioner: If it's okay with you, may I offer some suggestions and possible options?

Patient: Sure.

Practitioner: Looking at your insurance, you have Medicaid, and Medicaid will pay for transportation to doctors' appointments. You do need to call a Medicaid-approved service several days in advance to schedule. Also, ride services like Uber or Lyft may be cheaper than taxi and are usually readily available using an app. Would either of these work for you? (Open-ended question)

Patient: Well, I've got the money now for repairs, which is why I'm here today. I also just found out the county will be resuming bus service, but I still live far from a bus stop. So if my car breaks down again, both of those sound good. I would prefer the Medicaid option if I have enough time.

Practitioner: Okay, that sounds like a plan. If it's okay with you, I can refer you to the social worker to get the Medicaid transportation information.

Patient: Thank you.

MI can be used with health education strategies to enhance patient education. The next example demonstrates the elicit–provide–elicit (E-P-E) approach for exchanging information. This approach allows the practitioner to educate the patient and evoke patient responses, including feelings and emotions that could impact treatment.

Practitioner: As you know, we've been monitoring your blood pressure for the last 3 weeks, and it's been high every time you came in for a check-up. (Giving information)

Patient: Yes, the nurse told me.

Practitioner: What do you make of that? (Open-ended question)

Patient: Looks like I have high blood pressure. Do I need medication?

Practitioner: Yes, you may benefit from starting a medication to control your blood pressure. What, if anything, have you heard about high blood pressure? (Evoke)

Patient: Well, my father had it and had to take 3 or 4 pills a day. He died of a heart attack at age 65.

Practitioner: Your father had hypertension and was on daily medications, and you know it can lead to heart disease. What else do you remember about hypertension? (Evoke)

Patient: He had to watch his salt. He was always complaining about that. His legs swelled up.

Practitioner: He clearly had some difficulties managing his condition. (Reflection)

Patient: Yes, he didn't like taking his meds because of side effects, and he hated watching his diet.

Practitioner: How do you think you will handle medications and lifestyle changes? (Open-ended question)

Patient: Well, will I have to do all the things he was supposed to do?

Practitioner: Medication and lifestyle behaviors are key to managing high blood pressure. May I share some additional information that might be helpful to you about high blood pressure? (Asking permission to provide information/suggestions)

Patient: Yes, please.

Practitioner: [Explains the disease and need for medications, effects of hypertension on the heart, kidneys, etc.] (Provide) What do you make of all this? (Evoke)

Patient: Well, I want to live. It looks like I have to take a pill every day, watch my salt, lose weight, and exercise.

Practitioner: That's a lot to think about. What do you think would be most helpful to discuss more? (Open-ended question)

Patient: What about the medication? I hate to take another pill.

Practitioner: It's difficult to add another pill when you're already taking several pills for HIV, hepatitis C, and cholesterol treatment. Your blood pressure readings are very high, and medication is needed at this time to avoid serious complications. What concerns do you have about the medication? (Evoke)

Patient: Mainly I just don't want to take another pill and the side effects . . .

Practitioner: The pill is a reminder of having another diagnosis. (Reflection)

Patient: Yes, and I don't feel sick, so I hate to take another one and risk side effects.

Practitioner: You have your HIV and hepatitis C under control and feel healthy; you don't want to add another condition. We have lots of options for blood pressure medications now, and we can work together to get the one that works best for you. (Provide)

REFERENCES

1. Golin CE, Earp J, Tien HC, Stewart P, Porter C, Howie L. A 2-arm, randomized, controlled trial of a motivational interviewing-based intervention to improve adherence to antiretroviral therapy (ART) among patients failing or initiating ART. *J Acquir Immune Defic Syndr.* 2006;42(1):42–51.

2. Parsons JT, Golub SA, Rosof E, Holder C. Motivational interviewing and cognitive-behavioral intervention to improve HIV medication adherence among hazardous drinkers: a randomized controlled trial. *J Acquir Immune Defic Syndr.* 2007;46(4):443–445.

3. Goggin K, Gerkovich MM, Williams KB, et al. A randomized controlled trial examining the efficacy of motivational counseling with observed therapy for antiretroviral therapy adherence. *AIDS Behav.* 2013;17(6):1992–2001.

4. Holstad MM, Ofotokun I, Higgins M, Logwood S. The LIVE Network: a music-based messaging program to promote ART adherence self-management. *AIDS Behav.* 2013;17(9):2954–2962.

5. Golin CE, Earp JA, Grodensky CA, et al. Longitudinal effects of SafeTalk, a motivational interviewing-based program to improve safer sex practices among people living with HIV/AIDS. *AIDS Behav.* 2012;16(5):1182–1191.

6. Lovejoy TI, Heckman TG, Suhr JA, Anderson T, Heckman BD, France CR. Telephone-administered motivational interviewing reduces risky sexual behavior in HIV-positive late middle-age and older adults: a pilot randomized controlled trial. *AIDS Behav.* 2011;15(8):1623–1634.

7. Chen X, Murphy DA, Naar-king S, Parsons JT. A clinic-based motivational intervention improves condom use among subgroups of youth living with HIV. *J Adolesc Health.* 2011;49(2):193–198.

8. Naar-King S, Outlaw A, Green-Jones M, Wright K, Parsons JT. Motivational interviewing by peer outreach workers: a pilot randomized clinical trial to retain adolescents and young adults in HIV care. *AIDS Care*. 2009;21(7):868–873.

9. Naar-King S, Parsons JT, Murphy D, Kolmodin K, Harris DR; ATN 004 Protocol Team. A multisite randomized trial of a motivational intervention targeting multiple risks in youth living with HIV: initial effects on motivation, self-efficacy, and depression. *J Adolesc Health*. 2010;46(5):422–428.

10. Fisher JD, Cornman DH, Shuper PA, et al. HIV prevention counseling intervention delivered during routine clinical care reduces HIV risk behavior in HIV-infected South Africans receiving antiretroviral therapy: the Izindlela Zokuphila/Options for Health randomized trial. *J Acquir Immune Defic Syndr*. 2014;67(5):499–507.

11. Chariyeva Z, Golin CE, Earp JA, Maman S, Suchindran C, Zimmer C. The role of self-efficacy and motivation to explain the effect of motivational interviewing time on changes in risky sexual behavior among people living with HIV: a mediation analysis. *AIDS Behav*. 2013;17(2):813–823.

12. Chariyeva Z, Golin CE, Earp JA, Suchindran C. Does motivational interviewing counseling time influence HIV-positive persons' self-efficacy to practice safer sex?. *Patient Educ Couns*. 2012;87(1):101–107.

13. Murphy DA, Chen X, Naar-King S, Parsons JT. Alcohol and marijuana use outcomes in the Healthy Choices motivational interviewing intervention for HIV-positive youth. *AIDS Patient Care STDS*. 2012;26(2):95–100.

14. Rongkavilit C, Naar-king S, Wang B, et al. Motivational interviewing targeting risk behaviors for youth living with HIV in Thailand. *AIDS Behav*. 2013;17(6):2063–2074.

15. Lovejoy TI. Telephone-delivered motivational interviewing targeting sexual risk behavior reduces depression, anxiety, and stress in HIV-positive older adults. *Ann Behav Med*. 2012;44(3):416–421.

16. Holstad MM, Diiorio C, Kelley ME, Resnicow K, Sharma S. Group motivational interviewing to promote adherence to antiretroviral medications and risk reduction behaviors in HIV infected women. *AIDS Behav*. 2011;15(5):885–896.

17. Holstad MM, Essien JE, Ekong E, Higgins M, Teplinskiy I, Adewuyi MF. Motivational groups support adherence to antiretroviral therapy and use of risk reduction behaviors in HIV positive Nigerian women: a pilot study. *Afr J Reprod Health*. 2012;16(3):14–27.

18. Wagner CC, Ingersoll KS. *Motivational Interviewing in Groups*. New York, NY: Guilford Press; 2013.

19. Ingersoll KS, Farrell-Carnahan L, Cohen-Filipic J, et al. A pilot randomized clinical trial of two medication adherence and drug use interventions for HIV+ crack cocaine users. *Drug Alcohol Depend*. 2011;116(1–3):177–187.

20. Hasin DS, Aharonovich E, O'Leary A, et al. Reducing heavy drinking in HIV primary care: a randomized trial of brief intervention, with and without technological enhancement. *Addiction*. 2013;108(7):1230–1240.

21. Hasin DS, Aharonovich E, Greenstein E. HealthCall for the smartphone: technology enhancement of brief intervention in HIV alcohol dependent patients. *Addict Sci Clin Pract*. 2014;9:5.

22. Manuel JK, Lum PJ, Hengl NS, Sorensen JL. Smoking cessation interventions with female smokers living with HIV/AIDS: a randomized pilot study of motivational interviewing. *AIDS Care*. 2012;25(7):820–827.

16 Motivational Interviewing and Technology

Megan Mueller, Heidi Hutton,
Larry Chang, Lisa Hightow-Weidman,
Kelly Amy Knudtson, and K. Rivet Amico

With the growing use of mobile health (mHealth) technologies, MI has been used to guide the development and implementation of a number of interventions for people living with HIV. Over a decade ago, extensions of MI into mHealth approaches evolved using phone-based delivery of MI to replace or supplement in-person MI sessions.[1] While approaches used today vary in terms of aspects of technology leveraged, many technology-based projects adopt MI to guide principles of intervention delivery. Among interventions using MI to support HIV management, smartphones now allow for both delivery of brief MI sessions outside of clinical care settings,[2] text-based interactions, video-chat, app use and access to the Internet for Web-enabled intervention packages. In this chapter, we provide 3 examples of using MI in mHealth-based intervention approaches.

MI APPLIED TO A MHEALTH-ENABLED COMMUNITY HEALTH SCOUT INTERVENTION IN UGANDA

In a Lake Victoria fishing community of Rakai, Uganda, the mHealth Lakefolk Actively Keeping Engaged (mLAKE) trial used smartphones to guide community health workers' (CHW) delivery of MI-informed HIV prevention and care counseling (reference our trials protocol). The fishing community in Rakai is transient, the fishing are perilous, and hazardous alcohol use, sex work, and sexual transmission behaviors are common.[3] As a result, this area is a geographically defined hotspot with extremely high HIV transmission and prevalence (40%).[4] Resources and health system infrastructure, however, are modest, necessitating the use of community-based HIV interventions with CHWs to increase reach and maximize sustainability. To assist CHWs, a smartphone application was programmed (emocha Mobile Health Inc.,

Baltimore, MD, USA) to help CHWs navigate residents aged 15 years and older to HIV services. Using demographic and risk profile characteristics, (e.g., HIV-positive not in care or male, not circumcised), the algorithm determined which of 9 counseling modules and branches would be activated. The CHW followed the app to ask a series of approximately 10 tailored questions to ascertain the resident's information, motivation, and behavioral (IMB) skills to reduce risk of HIV or obtain HIV care. CHWs entered a checkbox on the smartphone to indicate that they had asked each question. CHWs were also trained in MI style to communicate with the residents.

As the app was programmed to be in MI style, all IMB-based counseling questions were open-ended. The app questions were prefaced with "what" or "how" versus use of the more confrontational and judgmental preface of "why." For example, "What do you know about taking antiretroviral therapy (ART) when you are pregnant?" Open-ended questions are a key strategy to support MI evocation and autonomy elements. The app questions were evocative to glean the residents' perspective (vs. presenting the CHW perspective) and to foster contemplation of the advantages of prevention or care behaviors. For example, "What are some benefits of using a condom?" To encourage autonomy, the app elicited residents' evaluation of potential facilitators and barriers to engaging services. "If you decided to seek circumcision, what would help you achieve this goal?" Additionally, the actual content of the app questions used other MI strategies to consider pros/cons and change rulers. Pros and cons questions were designed to develop discrepancy by querying benefits, concerns, and "not so good" outcomes that might result from pre-exposure prophylaxis (PrEP) for example. "What have been the not so good things that have happened or may happen by not getting PrEP?" Change rulers were incorporated by asking residents about their confidence in and readiness for action. Finally, to elicit potential change talk, the app queried intention to change and what would need to change for residents to want to achieve a target behavior.

Using smartphones to counsel provided structure and direction to the content of an IMB session. The app increased the likelihood that carefully crafted, nonjudgmental open-ended questions and all counseling content were reliably delivered, both of which can be challenging to maintain in interventions. Importantly, the app was complementary to the work of the CHWs. The CHWs provided the collaborative, empathic relationship through affirmations, reflections and summaries where the app could not. Notably, process results indicate that residents and CHWs reported that the smartphone was well accepted as part of the interview process. The major limitation of the app is the durability of the questions, which some residents found inflexible in follow-up visits. This is potentially modifiable in future deployments. The results of the trial will be available in 2020.

COMBINING MI-BASED STRATEGIES WITH ELECTRONIC DOSE MONITORING, VIDEO CONFERENCING, AND SMS-TRIGGERED ESCALATING REAL-TIME ADHERENCE ATN 152 STUDY TEAM

The Triggered Escalating Real-Time Adherence (TERA) study is a randomized clinical trial, which engages youth living with HIV who are failing ART, using MI strategies. This ongoing study examines the potential effect of this kind of intervention of viral outcomes after a 12-week intervention period and over time through week 48 of study participation.[5] Participants (youth aged 14–24 living with HIV who have detectable viral loads at study entry) are randomized to standard of care or 12 weeks of coach-facilitated adherence support through set video-conferenced sessions at point of care (baseline, 4 weeks, and 12 weeks) and electronic dose monitoring–triggered real-time SMS-based 2-way outreach.

Health coaches are located in one central location with all communication with participants through video conferencing and cell phone (SMS or phone calls). Coaches have diverse educational backgrounds and previous experiences with counseling and coaching. Each coach completes entry-level training in MI, in addition to specific training on the TERA intervention, which uses mixed medium approaches (e.g., pictures, drawing life spaces on shared screen, audio, video) as participants are guided through a planned sequence of topics. Part of these includes Next Step Counseling[6,7] specific to ART adherence, which relies heavily on MI-based spirit and strategies.

Within all communication with TERA participants, coaches strive to embody the MI spirit through collaborative problem-solving, evoking personal experiences and beliefs, and honoring patient autonomy.[8] Within video sessions, coaches engage with participants in conversations that explore their experiences living with HIV and barriers to taking daily medication. Coaches listen for change and sustain talk and work to create an adherence plan based on the ideas and experiences shared by the participant. During the latter 2 video sessions, coaches use the MI ruler[8] to rate and explore how important and how confident the participant feels taking their daily ART medications. Coaches guide participants in reflecting down and moving up the ruler.

Within SMS communication triggered by the electronic dose–monitoring device, most tenets of MI are possible to remain unchallenged. The TERA team developed strategies to promote partnership when dosing is not registered: participants receive a text asking "What's the plan? Reply (a) taking now (b) took already (c) taking later (d) other (e) pass" when 90 minutes pass from scheduled dose time without a registered opening of the electronic dose monitoring device. The "pass" option is available for use once every 7 days and gives youth the choice to not dose once weekly without further contact or questions from the coach. While certainly diverging from adherence, this pass allows youth to have autonomy. However, after use of the pass or in the event that the youth does not respond at all to the initial or subsequent SMS texts, respecting autonomy must be balanced with also wanting to promote partnership and maintain connections. In the case of continued declines to take ART doses, coaches escalate contact. For nonresponse, contact is attempted as well, through additional texts, phone calls, and using a contact tree. However, the team is also aware that this approach may work against collaboration and partnership, eroding respect for autonomy. To deal with this potential, the intervention adapted to include case-by-case procedures that allow coaches to adopt alternative approaches (e.g., spacing out contact attempts, shifting focus on contact attempts away from dosing and toward general health and well-being check-ins), which is documented in participant case notes.

As this trial is ongoing, unpacking the experiences of MI-based strategies from participants' and coaches' perspectives is not yet possible. Overall, use of MI for guiding spirit as well as strategies in delivery of this video-conferencing, electronic dose monitoring, and SMS coach–delivered intervention appears quite feasible. Tools used to monitoring fidelity and certain aspects of video-conference sessions that exemplify core, patient-centered, and MI features are also in use. Advised by the

Motivational Interviewing Treatment Integrity code, these adapted process evaluation tools will provide for opportunities to fully characterize the extent to which the spirit and principles used in the intervention and related material were actually embodied.

USE OF MI FOR PREP ADHERENCE IN YOUNG MSM VIA SMARTPHONE APP P3 STUDY TEAM

P3 (Prepared, Protected, emPowered) is a smartphone-based PrEP adherence app for HIV-uninfected young men who have sex with men (YMSM) and young transgender women who have sex with men (YTWSM) that utilizes social networking and game-based mechanics to improve PrEP adherence and persistence in PrEP care. P3 was developed to be engaging and age-appropriate and take advantage of technologies that are already embedded in the lives of YMSM and YTWSM. The accessibility, affordability, anonymity, and acceptability of smartphones make them the intervention medium of choice for youth engagement and a logical platform to deliver an adherence intervention targeting PrEP.[9] Further, smartphone interventions can overcome issues that impede engagement with in-person interventions such as transportation logistics, stigma, and confidentiality.

Despite the benefits of app-based interventions, maintaining engagement over time can be particularly challenging. Lack of rapport building may contribute to lower retention rates in technology-based interventions. Further, the available literature suggests that some tools, including technology-based tools, may be more beneficial to patient adherence when combined with education or counseling.[10-12] To investigate this possibility, the P3 team developed P3+. P3+ includes all of the functionality of P3 as well as an in-app texting portal that allows an adherence counselor to deliver integrated Next Step Counseling (iNSC). iNSC is a person-centered, discussion-based approach to promoting sexual health that focuses on needs related to making nonbiomedical prevention strategies as easy to use as possible in the context of one's current life and then moves into a discussion of decision making around PrEP and supporting PrEP use.[13] Principles of MI incorporated in iNSC include spirit (partnership, acceptance, compassion, and evocation), use of MI strategies to use exploration to identify change talk and foster autonomy in making small steps toward movement on continuum of change and maintenance. Although iNSC had been used to promote sexual health in a number of studies, the approach was delivered as a face to face, in person, or over telephone intervention. P3+ required real-time, in-app texting delivery.

P3's approach maintains the central tenet of iNSC and MI, using a client-centered, strengths-based discussion about sexual health and PrEP to assist individuals in identifying barriers and developing tailored strategies to address those barriers.

The P3 iNSC adaption was piloted in a 1-month field trial. Adherence counselors tested a variety of strategies integral to both iNSC and MI to understand which strategies translated to a text-based discussion, which needed adaption, and which did not work. The techniques and skills based on verbal communication (such as reframing, expressing empathy, and providing affirmations) were most easily translated to a texting discussion, while reflective listening statements, paraphrasing, and summarizing were not as well received during the field trial due to participants feeling like this caused unnecessary delays in counselor responses. Similarly, nonverbal communication (reading the participants body language or using silence as a tool), which is critical in in-person delivery of iNSC is not possible or does not function the same in a texting discussion. Quick responses were important for active engagement; silence or pausing made participants feel like the counselor was not there or the conversation was not "active." Adapting in-person counseling to an in-app texting platform requires more than just translation of talk to text. Prior to testing P3 in a 3-arm (P3, P3+, standard of care) nationwide randomized controlled trial, additional adaptations to the counseling protocol are being made to improve delivery and increase rapport building between the participant and counselor.

CONCLUSIONS

Although the 3 interventions presented use technology in unique ways, the adoption of MI as a manner in which patients can be fully engaged in interventions is consistent across them. The MI spirit promotes open exploration of ambivalence and use of change talk. Strategies vary in terms of whether discourse is centered on SMS texts, phone conversation, or in-person discussions, but all leverage MI strategies and conceptualizations of patients as their own agents of change in support of HIV prevention and treatment strategies.

REFERENCES

1. Aharonovich E, Greenstein E, O'Leary A, Johnston B, Seol SG, Hasin DS. HealthCall: technology-based extension of motivational interviewing to reduce non-injection drug use in HIV primary care patients—a pilot study. *AIDS Care.* 2012;24(12):1461–1469.
2. Aharonovich E, Stohl M, Cannizzaro D, Hasin D. HealthCall delivered via smartphone to reduce co-occurring drug and alcohol use in HIV-infected adults: A randomized pilot trial. *J Subst Abuse Treat.* 2017;83:15–26.
3. Lubega M, Nakyaanjo N, Nansubuga S, et al. Understanding the socio-structural context of high HIV transmission in kasensero fishing community, South Western Uganda. *BMC Public Health.* 2015;15(1):1033.
4. Chang LW, Grabowski MK, Ssekubugu R, et al. Heterogeneity of the HIV epidemic in agrarian, trading, and fishing communities in Rakai, Uganda: an observational epidemiological study. *Lancet HIV.* 2016;3(8):e388–e396.
5. Amico KR, Dunlap A, Dallas R, et al. Triggered escalating real-time adherence intervention to promote rapid HIV viral suppression among youth living with HIV failing antiretroviral therapy: protocol for a triggered escalating real-time adherence intervention. *JMIR Res Protoc.* 2019;8(3):e11416.
6. Amico K, McMahan V, Goicochea P, et al. Supporting study product use and accuracy in self-report in the iPrEx study: next step counseling and neutral assessment. *AIDS Behav.* 2012;16(5):1243–1259.
7. Amico KR, Mansoor LE, Corneli A, Torjesen K, van der Straten A. Adherence support approaches in biomedical HIV prevention trials: experiences, insights and future directions from four multisite prevention trials. *AIDS Behav.* 2013;17(6):2143–2155.
8. Rollnick S, Miller WR, Butler CC, Aloia MS. *Motivational Interviewing in Health Care: Helping Patients Change Behavior.* New York, NY: Taylor & Francis; 2008.
9. Campbell JL, Quincy C, Osserman J, Pedersen OK. Coding in-depth semistructured interviews: problems of unitization and intercoder reliability and agreement. *Sociol Method Res.* 2013;42(3):294–320.

10. McPherson-Baker S, Malow RM, Penedo F, Jones DL, Schneiderman N, Klimas NG. Enhancing adherence to combination antiretroviral therapy in non-adherent HIV-positive men. *AIDS Care*. 2000;12(4):399–404.

11. Simoni JM, Chen WT, Huh D, et al. A preliminary randomized controlled trial of a nurse-delivered medication adherence intervention among HIV-positive outpatients initiating antiretroviral therapy in Beijing, China. *AIDS Behav*. 2011;15(5):919–929.

12. Mannheimer SB, Morse E, Matts JP, et al. Sustained benefit from a long-term antiretroviral adherence intervention: results of a large randomized clinical trial. *J Acquir Immune Defic Syndr*. 2006;43(Suppl 1):S41–S47.

13. Amico KR, Miller J, Balthazar C, et al. Integrated Next Step Counseling (iNSC) for sexual health and PrEP use among young men who have sex with men: implementation and observations from ATN110/113. *AIDS Behav*. 2019;23(7):1812–1823.

SECTION V
ETHICS

17 Ethical Challenges in the Applications of Motivational Interviewing in HIV Care

Isra Black and Lisa Forsberg

INTRODUCTION

Miller and Rollnick[1p12] define motivational interviewing (MI) as:

A collaborative, goal-oriented style of communication with particular attention to the language of change. It is designed to strengthen personal motivation for and commitment to a specific goal [or target behavior] by eliciting and exploring the person's own reasons for change within an atmosphere of acceptance and compassion.

On this definition, MI is an intervention administered by one person that is designed to facilitate another person's behavior change. The available evidence suggests that MI can be effective in bringing about behavior change in clients.[2-5] On the one hand, the fact that MI aims to and can change behavior might be thought morally desirable. Change may be good for a client, or good in general. And if a particular behavior change is desirable, MI may be an effective means to this end. For example, it seems good for individuals to reduce harmful and hazardous drinking and hence appropriate to use MI to facilitate this change. On the other hand, the fact that MI can be effective in altering motivation and behavior may give rise to concerns about its moral permissibility and that of its applications.[6-8] For instance, Miller and Rollnick[1,9] have consistently cited sales as an example of a setting in which MI-type interventions would be ethically inappropriate.

In this chapter, we engage with ethical challenges of using MI and MI-based interventions in HIV care (for brevity, we use MI to refer to both MI and MI-based interventions). First, we briefly describe the technical and relational components of MI and discuss 2 general ethical worries in respect of MI use: (i) that the relation component fails to provide sufficient ethical action guidance and (ii) that the technical component fails to safeguard against manipulation. Second, we consider these ethical concerns in the context of HIV care, specifically in relation to pre-exposure prophylaxis (PrEP), medication adherence, and disclosure of HIV/AIDS diagnosis/prognosis.

TWO ETHICAL WORRIES ABOUT MI

In this section, we briefly describe the components of MI. We draw on these components in the subsequent discussion of 2 ethical concerns in respect of MI use: (i) ethical action guidance and (ii) safeguards against manipulation.

As a caveat to what follows, while we argue that MI practitioners and institutions considering adopting MI interventions should be aware of these ethical issues, it is important to recognize the need for comparative ethical analysis. The use of MI requires consideration against possible alternatives, including treatment-as-usual approaches, delegation to individual practitioner discretion, or doing nothing. Even taking into account the ethical concerns about MI we discuss in the following text, MI may be ethically preferable to these alternatives, all things considered.

By way of clarification of terminology, we understand by "permissible" and "permissibility" that an option is ethically appropriate. The claim that an option is ethically permissible etc. is weaker than the claim that an option is ethically obligatory or required.

The Components of MI

MI can be described in terms of its technical and relational components, and the core skills that operationalize the former.

The technical component of MI involves 4 "sequential and recursive" overlapping processes: *engagement, focusing, evocation*, and *planning*.[1pp25,26] *Engagement* involves the practitioner seeking to "establish a helpful connection and working relationship" with the client.[1p26] *Focusing* involves selection of a conversational target, such as quitting smoking. Through the *evocation* process, the MI practitioner engages with the conversational target by "selectively eliciting and reinforcing the client's own arguments and motivations for change"—change talk, while taking care not to evoke sustain talk that favors current behavior.[10p28] MI is unlike "traditional conceptions of client-centred counselling," therefore, in that through focusing and evocation, it is "consciously goal-oriented, in having intentional direction toward change."[10pp27,28] The fourth technical process of MI is *planning*: the development of commitment to change and formulation of a plan for its achievement.

The counterpart to the technical component of MI is its relational, person-centered spirit, which consists of 4 interrelated practitioner dispositions: *partnership, acceptance, compassion*, and *evocation*.[1] *Partnership* requires the practitioner to see the MI encounter as an "active collaboration between experts" in which the "interviewer seeks to create a positive interpersonal atmosphere that is conducive to change but not coercive."[1p15] Second, *acceptance* requires (i) recognition of the client's *absolute worth*; (ii) *empathy*, that is, "an active interest in and effort to understand the other's internal perspective"; (iii) respect for the client's *autonomy* and power of decision in respect of behavior change; and (iv) *affirmation* of the client's strengths and efforts.[1pp16,17] Third, *compassion* enjoins the MI practitioner to "to pursue the welfare and best interests of the other."[1] Fourth, the MI spirit requires *evocation* of the client's own motivation and resources to change.

Four core skills operationalize the technical and relational components of MI: *open-ended questions, affirmation, reflections,* and *summaries.*[1] *Open-ended questions* promote collaboration between the parties and invite the client to reflect and elaborate. *Affirmation* involves active acknowledgement of the client's positive dispositions. Through *reflections* that attempt (selectively) to clarify meaning, the MI practitioner offers an opportunity to the client to replay her thoughts and feelings. *Summaries* are reflections that collate the client's utterances; these may help to establish alliance, identify themes, transition between the technical processes, and provide the client an opportunity to add meaning and clarity for themselves and the practitioner.

Ethical Action Guidance and Safeguards against Manipulation

In this section, we discuss the adequacy of the ethical action guidance and safeguards against manipulation theorized to exist within the relational and technical components of MI, respectively. We argue that the relational component of MI alone cannot guide against the use of MI for inappropriate target behaviors. In addition, it is implausible to think that the technical component of MI could never have a manipulative effect. It is necessary, in our view, to consider factors external to the method of MI to establish the ethical permissibility of its use in a particular setting.

Miller and Rollnick[10] argue that "it would be unethical, for example, to attempt to use MI as a way to sell a product, fill private treatment beds, or obtain consent to participate in research." What is there to prevent MI use in ethically inappropriate settings or to ethically inappropriate ends, for example, in sales and advertising or to encourage migrants to coalesce to their impending deportation? A possible response to this question is that elements of the MI spirit, namely, *respect for autonomy* or *compassion*, provide ethical action guidance against such use.

It might be thought that respect for autonomy can provide sufficient guidance for ethical MI practice. In this sense, MI use in pursuit of a behavioral outcome might be grounded on the claim that an individual desires that outcome or that people in general desire that outcome. However, respect for autonomy is both too broad and too narrow a criterion for ethical action guidance. It is too broad because what individuals' desires do not necessarily determine their best interests to the extent that if one can show that a client desires an outcome, this dispels all ethical concern. For example, a bookmaker might respect a thrill-seeking individual's autonomy by using MI to encourage them to stake bets with the possibility of huge gains yet probability of significant losses. Nevertheless, we might be uneasy about the use of MI to this end. Respect for autonomy is also too narrow because it might be possible for things that are not desired to be good for individuals. For example, we argue in the following discussion that it may be permissible to use MI to direct toward disclosure of HIV transmission risk, even if an individual has a preference not to disclose.

One might instead attempt to use compassion as the criterion for determining ethical appropriate target behaviors. Miller and Rollnick[1p20] argue that compassion precludes the practice of MI "in pursuit of self-interest." Conceived in this way, the compassion criterion may be able to ward against some of worst applications of MI. For example, it might rule out using MI to exploit an individual's thrill-seeking nature for profit by encouraging gambling. However, compassion construed as the disavowal of self-interest may still permit too much, ethically speaking. For example, we grant, like Miller and Rollnick[1p14] that "'promotion of others' welfare is . . . one motivation that draws people into helping professions." But the fact that an MI practitioner is well-intentioned, or acts with the client's best interests at heart, does not rule out the seeking of inappropriate target behaviors. The conception of compassion within MI spirit is practitioner-focused. However, practitioners may be mistaken in their view of a client's best interest. For example, an MI-trained oncologist might consider that an additional cycle of chemotherapy is in their client's best interests and direct toward this outcome, when many factors count against curative treatment, from the client's own perspective or more objectively.

It might be argued that ethical action guidance is not provided by the use of respect for autonomy or compassion alone, but together. However, respect for autonomy and compassion may conflict, which may lead to difficulty in knowing whether an MI intervention is ethically permissible. Consider a version of the previously noted cancer case, in which the MI-trained oncologist is correct that a further cycle of chemotherapy would be in their client's best interest, but the client expresses an autonomous wish not to undergo the treatment. If the practitioner was to use MI to seek consent to treatment, this would be paternalistic. Paternalism by definition involves a failure to respect an individual's autonomy in pursuit of their well-being[11] It is often thought to be (highly) morally problematic in healthcare settings. Yet, according to the MI spirit, it would be an open question whether seeking consent in this scenario would be an appropriate target behavior, given the tension between respect for autonomy and compassion. As such, respect for autonomy and compassion together fail to give sufficient ethical action guidance.

One might accept that one cannot derive before the fact ethical action guidance from MI spirit. However, it might be argued that this is unnecessary or irrelevant given the way in which the technical component of MI is theorized to operate. Miller and Rollnick[1chapter 2,p14] argue that "[u]nless the change is in some way consistent with the client's own goals or values, there is no basis for MI to work." This might be interpreted, despite what Miller and Rollnick claim elsewhere, to permit MI use for any target behavior, since MI will be effective only if the outcome is consistent with the client's goals or values, and if this is the case, the intervention is ethically permissible. However, this seems to be very ethically undemanding.

In any event, we think that the claim about the technical component of MI such that it works only when a client possesses a goal or value that aligns with the target behavior is implausible. We have suggested elsewhere that evocation of any change talk, that is, "the selective reinforcement of any utterances, not just those which align with core values and beliefs," may influence behavior.[7] Black and Helgason[8] argue: "The idea is that the evocation of talk that favours a distinct outcome may distort or pervert the interviewee's decision-making processes by minimising potentially cogent reasons against that choice. In so doing, MI potentially inhibits the ability of the interviewee to reach an adequately deliberated decision." The upshot of this argument is that we cannot be confident that MI is never problematically manipulative, that is, that MI never involves intentional conduct that "infringes upon the autonomy of the victim by subverting and insulting their decision-making powers."[12] It is not clear that when MI use is successful in bringing about behavior change, it always respects client autonomy.

Where does the foregoing leave us in respect of the ethics of MI? First, we argue that the respect for autonomy or compassion requirements of MI spirit do not provide sufficient action guidance for ethical MI use. Second, we argue that MI may be problematically manipulative. In respect of the first concern, we cannot rely on the relational component of MI alone to ward against practice that seeks unethical behavioral outcomes. We must confront this challenge head on, through consideration of factors external to the method of MI to establish the ethical permissibility of its applications. In particular, we ought not to outsource or delegate the determination of ethical permissibility to individual MI practitioners or institutions. In respect of the second concern, we believe that it is necessary to accept the risk that MI is manipulative and engage in frank discussion about when manipulation might be justified given the benefits to be gained from a given application of MI.

In general, there may not be a one-size-fits-all answer to whether an application of MI is ethically permissible. In all cases, careful consideration of factors such as the expected benefit of the intervention to the client or others, the degree to which the intervention is likely to be respectful of autonomy, and social and institutional factors that may affect benefit or respect for autonomy etc. will be required.

ETHICAL MI USE IN HIV CARE

In this section, we tentatively discuss the ethical permissibility of MI use in 3 contexts relevant to HIV care: PrEP, medication adherence, and disclosure of HIV/AIDS diagnosis/prognosis. Our framework for discussion of these issues may be relevant to other applications of MI in HIV care. However, we stress that the substantive conclusions we draw may not transfer directly to other MI applications.

PrEP

PrEP involves HIV-negative individuals following a course of daily antiretroviral medication to reduce the risk of infection. Clinical trials have shown PrEP to reduce the risk of HIV transmission significantly,[13,14] with possible attendant health and psychological benefits.[15] However, there exist possible negative health effects[13,14] of PrEP, as well as social stigma around its use in certain populations.[16] Since individuals may be ambivalent about the use of PrEP or these latter reasons, it may seem a good candidate for an MI intervention. Indeed, research into MI-based PrEP interventions is underway.[17]

Would it be ethically permissible to employ MI to help clients resolve ambivalence in the direction of PrEP use? At first blush, it seems straightforwardly ethically permissible to seek PrEP use as a behavioral outcome. PrEP is clearly good for a great majority of individuals who take it, and there is a population health interest in reducing the number of HIV infections. The risk of manipulation, that is, the risk that some individuals who do not wish to use PrEP might have their autonomy infringed by MI, will vary according to local acceptance of PrEP. However, it is arguable that this risk is acceptable in general given the benefits both to individuals who do not have a prior desire for PrEP and the community at large.

That being said, PrEP is perhaps a good example of the necessity to consider very carefully the ethical permissibility of MI interventions in context. It is possible that PrEP uptake gives rise to community-level risk compensation, or "prevention optimism," that is, increased risk tolerance toward condomless sex among non-PrEP users in virtue of "a belief that they are indirectly protected from HIV because of the greater use of PrEP by others."[18,19] In addition, there are possible non-HIV-related negative consequences from condomless sex, such as the increased risk of certain sexually transmitted infections. These factors potentially make PrEP use less beneficial to individuals who use it and possibly pit the benefits of PrEP for users against population health. That is not to say that the use of MI to help resolve ambivalence in favor of PrEP use would be ethically impermissible. Rather the permissibility of any such intervention depends on the existence and availability of counterpart measures such as public education campaigns, accessible sexual health services, and interventions (including those that are MI-based) aimed at increasing medication adherence.

Medication Adherence

Antiretroviral medication adherence is key to the prophylactic effect of PrEP and reduction in viral load among individuals living with HIV/AIDS. However, some individuals may experience difficulty maintaining high levels of medication adherence or be ambivalent about it. For example, an individual may experience a tension between concern for their own health (because of nonadherence) as well as that for others (through transmission risk) and responsibilities toward others arising from work or family circumstances. Or an individual may experience negative side effects of antiretroviral therapy (ART) that disincentivize medication adherence. Again, MI would seem to be a good candidate intervention for resolving ambivalence in the direction of adherence.

Similar to our argument in respect of PrEP use, we submit that medication adherence clearly is good for individuals taking PrEP or ART and good for the community at large, and any risk of manipulation is acceptable for these reasons.

However, MI use for medication adherence among individuals with HIV may be more complicated than initially appears, to the extent that respect for a client's inconsistent ART adherence may implicitly involve taking a stance on the potential trade-off between viral load and drug resistance. Reduced ART adherence is associated with increased risk of drug resistance,[20,21] and reduced ART adherence correlates with increased viral load.[22] While we are not certain, it is possible that it may ethically appropriate in respect of some clients to switch target behavior to a decision about whether to take ART at all, because it ought to be for the client to decide how to manage this trade-off. In addition, in the face of confirmed opposition to ART adherence, it may be ethically permissible to direct clients toward (perhaps temporary) nonuse of ART, if inconsistent use carries a significant risk of drug resistance and HIV transmission.[23]

Disclosure of Diagnosis and Prognosis

Disclosure of diagnosis may be a difficult matter for individuals living with HIV/AIDS, in particular because of the severe stigma and discrimination attached to HIV-positive status in many communities. In this section, we discuss the ethical issues arising in 3 potentially overlapping contexts in which a practitioner might consider MI use: disclosure of transmission risk, disclosure to close personal relations, and disclosure at the end of life. In each case, the ethical question is, in our view, whether to use MI in the direction of disclosure or to use "decisional balance" MI to aid a client to take a decision about disclosure.

So far as disclosure of transmission risk is concerned, for example, to sexual partners or to IV drug users through needle sharing, we take the view that it is invariably permissible to direct toward disclosure. It is difficult to see how knowing exposure of others to risk of HIV/AIDS infection could be morally justifiable, even taking into account the fact that disclosure may make the client worse off. And in many jurisdictions serious criminal law penalties attach to intentional or reckless HIV transmission. To approach disclosure of transmission risk as a decisional balance issue would give too much credence to nondisclosure of transmission risk being a legitimate choice.

In disclosure contexts in which transmission risk is absent, it may be less clear that directional MI is ethically appropriate. In respect of disclosure to close personal relations, it might be thought that disclosure could be beneficial to the client, because "[p]atients who have a support network function better than those who are isolated."[24p6] However, as the US Department of Health and Human Services[24p6] notes in its clinical guideline "patients fears of disclosure are often well founded." Close personal relations may not respond with support. Moreover, clients may fear stigma and discrimination in virtue of disclosure, particularly if their HIV status becomes widely known within their community. And we should not discount that in some populations, the risk of serious harms, such as personal violence and even death, can follow the disclosure of HIV-positive status. Of course, in other communities, HIV stigma is tricky to negotiate. By recognizing that stigma counts as a reason against disclosure, the MI practitioner may be seen to reinforce or validate it. And arguably one way to combat HIV stigma is to increase the visibility of seropositive status within a community. Nevertheless, we think in general that decisional balance is the appropriate MI stance to take toward disclosure when transmission risk is absent.

A final specific disclosure context that may be relevant to individuals living with HIV/AIDS is end-of-life care. As Black and Helgason[8] note,

individuals may be ambivalent about disclosure of end-of-life diagnosis/prognosis to loved-ones. . . . On the one hand, an individual may wish to disclose so that loved-ones can prepare for bereavement, or in order to have support while dying, itself essential to good palliative care; on the other hand, an individual may wish not to disclose out of a desire to maintain hope of recovery, or to spare loved-ones trauma . . . or because of estrangement or other complicating interpersonal factors.

MI practitioners may consider using MI to facilitate disclosure of end-of-life diagnosis and prognosis by clients to mitigate the potential negative health effects of unprepared bereavement.[8] Black and Helgason[8] argue that whether disclosure is in an individual's best interests is likely to depend on her "wishes and preferences and her situation" and that it is difficult to gauge the risk that MI use would be manipulative in this setting. These factors point toward decisional balance MI being the ethically appropriate approach in respect of disclosure at the end of life.

However, Black and Helgason[8] also argue that "insofar as non-directive MI may be more difficult to learn and [to] practise than directional MI . . . it may be ethically permissible, all things considered, to have disclosure as the target behavior of an MI-based [disclosure] intervention." The idea is that it may be unethical to gain client consent to a decisional balance MI intervention, yet fail to deliver it, in virtue of the "still higher level of clinical skilfulness [required compared to] the directive variety of counselling, because [in decisional balance MI] one must avoid inadvertently tipping the scales in one direction or the other."[9] Thus, while having disclosure as the target behavior for an MI intervention may not clearly be in a client's best interests and also potentially manipulate them into disclosure, it may be ethically preferable for practitioners to be open with clients that they favor disclosure when the alternative is infringing client autonomy by failing to provide a decisional balance MI intervention. This argument applies equally to disclosure to close personal relations outside of the end-of-life setting.

CONCLUSION

In this chapter we described the relational and technical components of MI. We argued that these components fail to provide sufficient ethical action guidance and safeguards against manipulation, respectively. We subsequently considered the ethical permissibility of MI use in HIV care in respect of PrEP, medication adherence, and disclosure of HIV/AIDS diagnosis and prognosis. It is necessary to consider factors external to the method of MI to establish the ethical permissibility of its applications, including the expected benefit of the intervention to the client or others, the degree to which the intervention is likely to be respectful of autonomy, and social and institutional factors that may affect benefit or respect for autonomy.

REFERENCES

1. Miller WR, Rollnick S. *Motivational Interviewing, Helping People Change.* New York, NY: Guilford Press; 2012.
2. Hettema J, Steele J, Miller WR. Motivational interviewing. *Annu Rev Clin Psychol.* 2005;1:91–111.
3. Lundahl B, Moleni T, Burke BL, et al. Motivational interviewing in medical care settings: a systematic review and meta-analysis of randomized controlled trials. *Patient Educ Couns.* 2013;93(2):157–168.
4. Lundahl BW, Kunz C, Brownell C, Tollefson D, Burke BL. A meta-analysis of motivational interviewing: twenty-five years of empirical studies. *RSWP.* 2010;20(2):137–116.
5. Rubak S, Sandbaek A, Lauritzen T, Christensen B. Motivational interviewing: a systematic review and meta-analysis. *Br J Gen Pract.* 2005;55(513):305–312.
6. Miller WR. Motivational interviewing: III. On the ethics of motivational intervention. *Behav Cogn Psychother.* 1994;22(02):111–123.
7. Black I, Forsberg L. Would it be ethical to use motivational interviewing to increase family consent to deceased solid organ donation? *J Med Ethics.* 2014;40(1):63–68.
8. Black I, Helgason AR. Using motivational interviewing to facilitate death talk in end-of-life care: an ethical analysis. *BMC Palliat Care.* 2018;17(1):51.
9. Miller WR, Rollnick S. *Motivational Interviewing, Preparing People to Change Addictive Behavior.* New York, NY: Guilford Press; 2002.
10. Miller WR, Rollnick S. Ten things that motivational interviewing is not. *Behav Cogn Psychother.* 2009;37(2):129–140.
11. Dworkin G. *The Theory and Practice of Autonomy.* Cambridge, England: Cambridge University Press; 1988. doi:10.1017/CBO9780511625206
12. Wilkinson TM. Nudging and manipulation. *Polit Stud.* 2013;61(2):341–355.

13. Choopanya K, Martin M, Suntharasamai P, et al. Antiretroviral prophylaxis for HIV infection in injecting drug users in Bangkok, Thailand (the Bangkok Tenofovir Study): a randomised, double-blind, placebo-controlled phase 3 trial. *Lancet.* 2013;381(9883):2083–2090.

14. Grant RM, Lama JR, Anderson PL, et al. Preexposure chemoprophylaxis for HIV prevention in men who have sex with men. *N Engl J Med.* 2010;363(27):2587–2599. doi:10.1056/NEJMoa1011205

15. Holt M, Lea T, Bear B, et al. Trends in attitudes to and the use of HIV pre-exposure prophylaxis by Australian gay and bisexual men, 2011–2017: implications for further implementation from a diffusion of innovations perspective. *AIDS Behav.* 2019;23(7):1939–1950.

16. Calabrese SK, Underhill K. How stigma surrounding the use of HIV preexposure prophylaxis undermines prevention and pleasure: a call to destigmatize "Truvada whores." *Am J Public Health.* 2015;105(10):1960–1964.

17. John SA, Rendina HJ, Starks TJ, Grov C, Parsons JT. Decisional balance and contemplation ladder to support interventions for HIV pre-exposure prophylaxis uptake and persistence. *AIDS Patient Care STDS.* 2019;33(2):67–78.

18. Holt M, Lea T, Mao L, et al. Community-level changes in condom use and uptake of HIV pre-exposure prophylaxis by gay and bisexual men in Melbourne and Sydney, Australia: results of repeated behavioural surveillance in 2013-17. *Lancet HIV.* 2018;5(8):e448–e456.

19. Holt M, Murphy DA. Individual versus community-level risk compensation following preexposure prophylaxis of HIV. *Am J Public Health.* 2017;107(10):1568–1571.

20. Gardner EM, Hullsiek KH, Telzak EE, et al. Antiretroviral medication adherence and class- specific resistance in a large prospective clinical trial. *AIDS.* 2010;24(3):395–403.

21. Gardner EM, Sharma S, Peng G, et al. Differential adherence to combination antiretroviral therapy is associated with virological failure with resistance. *AIDS.* 2008;22(1):75–82.

22. Genberg BL, Wilson IB, Bangsberg DR, et al. Patterns of antiretroviral therapy adherence and impact on HIV RNA among patients in North America. *AIDS.* 2012;26(11):1415–1423

23. Wertheim JO, Oster AM, Johnson JA, et al. Transmission fitness of drug-resistant HIV revealed in a surveillance system transmission network. *Virus Evol.* 2017;3(1):vex008.

24. US Department of Health and Human Services. Guide for HIV/AIDS clinical care. https://hab.hrsa.gov/sites/default/files/hab/clinical-quality-management/2014guide.pdf. Published April 2014.

Index